STOP MANIPULATING ME!

Identifying Narcissism,
Disarming A Narcissist
& Overcoming Narcissistic Abuse

By Lisa Howard

Copyright© 2019 by Lisa Howard - All rights reserved.

Copyright: No part of this publication may be reproduced without written permission from the author, except by a reviewer who may quote brief passages or reproduce illustrations in a review with appropriate credits; nor may any part of this book be reproduced, stored in a retrieval system, or transmitted in any form or by any means – electronic, mechanical, photocopying, recording, or other – without prior written permission of the copyright holder.

The trademarks are used without any consent, and the publication of the trademark is without permission or backing by the trademark owner. All trademarks and brands within this book are for clarifying purposes only and are owned by the owners themselves.

Disclaimer: The information in this book is not to be used as professional medical advice and is not meant to treat or diagnose medical problems. The information presented should be used in combination with guidance from a competent professional person.

The information in this book is true and complete to the best of our knowledge. All recommendations are made without guarantee on the part of the author. It is the sole responsibility of the reader to educate and train in the use of all or any specialized equipment that may be used or referenced in this book that could cause harm or injury to the user or applicant. The author disclaims any liability in connection with the use of this information. References are provided for informational purposes only and do not constitute endorsement of any websites or other sources. Readers should be aware that the websites listed in this book may change.

First Printing, 2019 - Printed in the United States of America

TABLE OF CONTENTS

Introduction	1
All You Need to Know About Narcissism	5
What Is It?	5
4 Little-Known Causes of Narcissism	7
The Science of Narcissism	14
60-Second Narcissism Quiz	16
When Does This Become a *Real* Issue?	19
8 Surprising Narcissism Facts	27
25 Proven Steps to Discover Narcissism	31
An Ideal Target	31
What a Narcissist Wants?	33
The Effect on Me	34
6 Secret Tools Narcissists Use for Emotional Manipulation	35
5 Subtle Signs to Look Out For	37
10 Unexplored Ways Narcissism Affects You	39
8 Time-Tested Tactics to Overcome Narcissism	61
Glossary	81
FAQs	89
Conclusion	93
About the Author	97

INTRODUCTION

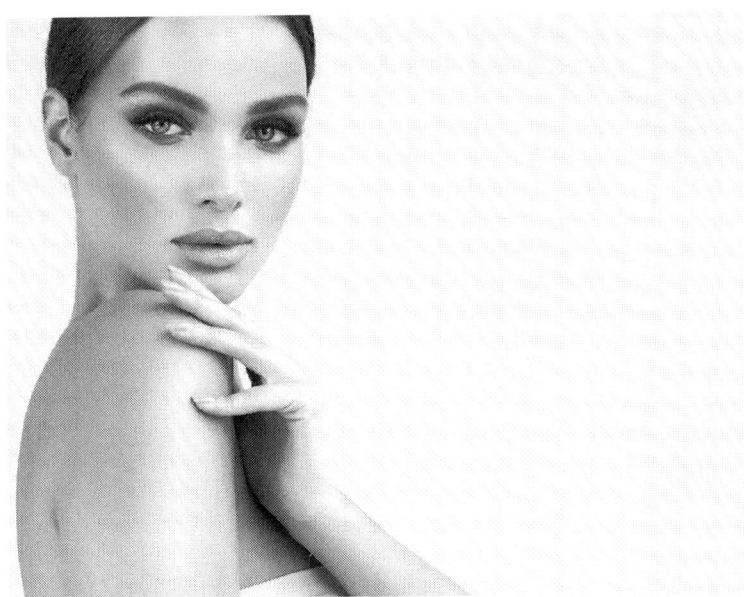

The word *narcissism* comes from the Greek myth of Narcissus, which is a metaphor of self-absorption and the inability to love another person.

Psychology Today (at *psychologytoday.com/basics/narcissism*) defines narcissism as *"a personality disorder in which there is a long-term pattern of abnormal behavior characterized by exaggerated feelings of self-importance, an excessive need for admiration, and a lack of understanding of others' feelings."*

Below are **some signs to look out for if you're trying to identify a narcissist**:

- An exaggerated idea of their own importance.
- A feeling of entitlement that drives the need for constant admiration.
- The need to be treated as superior at all times.

- A hyper focus on personal abilities and achievements.
- A chronic drive to pursue power and success.
- A belief that they are inherently better than everyone else.
- Taking control of every conversation.
- The expectation of special treatment when it isn't earned, deserved.
- Using others to get what they want, where they want to be.
- Unwilling to see the emotions or needs of anyone else.
- A feeling of envy for others; the belief everyone envies them.
- An arrogant or haughty personality, acting pretentious and boastful.
- A hyper focus on acquiring only "the best" of anything they own.

Does this sound familiar to you? Maybe it's a statement that you can personally relate to, or it reminds you of someone you know. Since it's estimated that 6% of the population suffers from this problem, it's likely that you do! Either way, this is the book for you. The following chapters will help you to understand the core of the problem, not just the symptoms of it. This knowledge of what *causes* someone to become narcissistic will help you to overcome it. You'll learn how to separate yourself from the problem and to become less susceptible to a narcissist's control.

If this sounds like something you believe will help you, then please read on for all the tips you'll need to start taking back some of the control in your life, leading to a much brighter future.

The traits leading to a diagnosis include:

- Reacting to criticism with humiliation, anger, or shame.
- Taking advantage of others to benefit yourself; for example, to reach your own goals.
- Exaggerating one's own self-importance and talent.
- Unrealistic fantasies of success, power, intelligence, beauty, or even romance.

STOP MANIPULATING ME!

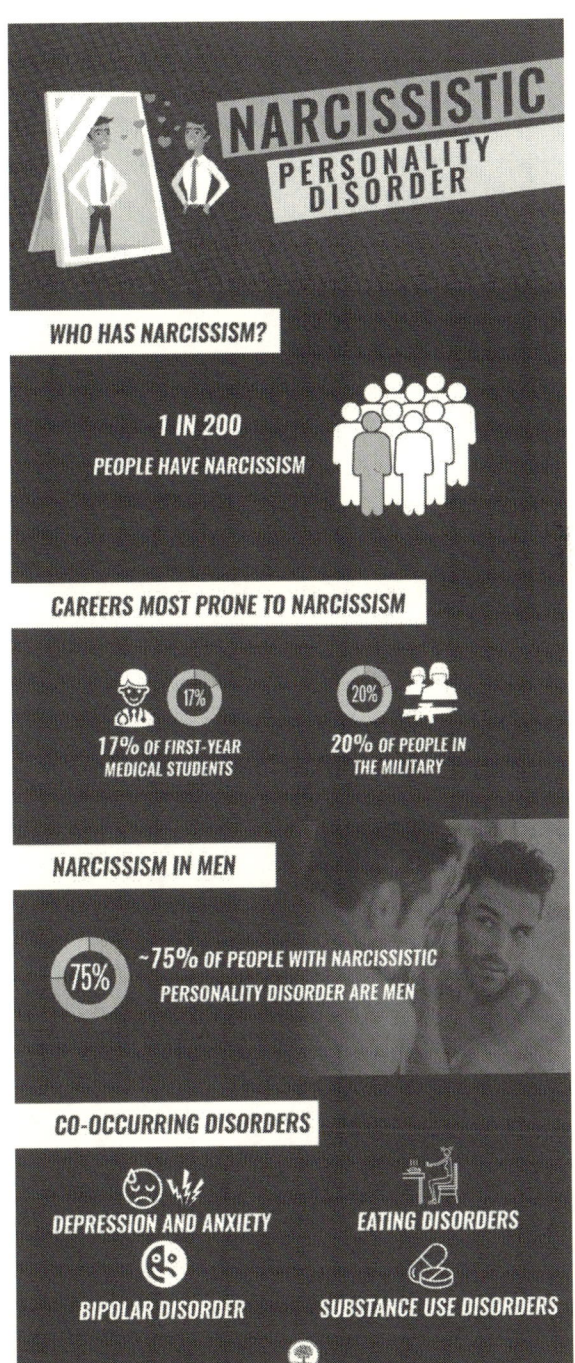

ALL YOU NEED TO KNOW ABOUT NARCISSISM

WHAT IS IT?

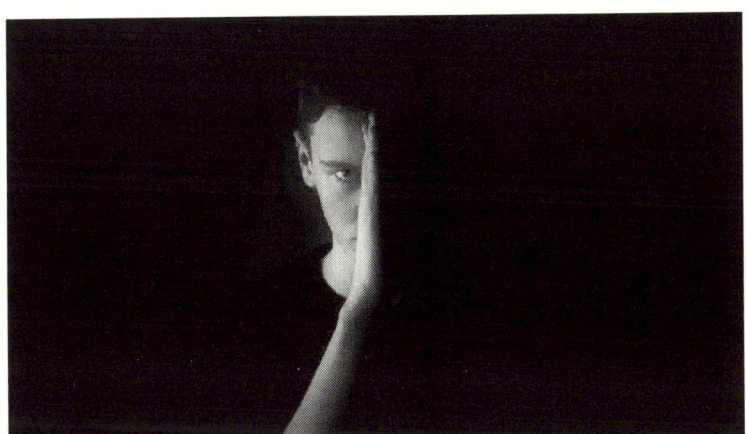

So, we explained the clinical definition of narcissism in the introduction, along with some traits that you might find in someone who suffers from this personality disorder, but what does that really tell us? It lets us know that *now* someone has become selfish and self-important, but it doesn't give any clue as to *how* someone became that way.

None of us are born with narcissistic tendencies; it's something that comes with life.

Understanding *how* someone develops this trait is the first step to make a difference to them, yourself, and everyone else in their life.

It is believed that narcissism comes from the idea that the perpetrator believes their needs must be met first and foremost before anything else.

However, a study by **Psychology Today** (at <u>psychologytoday.com/blog/shame/201211/narcissism-and-other-defenses-against-shame</u>) suggests that the tendencies come from a place of shame. The author of the research suggests that the feelings associated with narcissism are a defense mechanism. It's a reaction people have, trying to display the beauty on the outside to hide ugly on the inside, trying to cover up some negative emotions that they feel inside.

This might be something that you already know, especially, if you suffer from narcissism or you live with someone who has it. Maybe you know they have emotions they're struggling with or some past shame. You just didn't realize that it linked to these tendencies.

However...a new study presented at **Lucky Otter** (at <u>luckyottershaven.com</u>) suggests that the tendencies actually come from a place of envy. The creator of the study *"believes envy is a primitive form of hatred. Envy is, of course, a defense against toxic shame."*

Still, **this all links to shame**, and since many extensive scientific studies agree with this, this is an area we will be exploring more in the content of this book. Shame can manifest itself in a number of different ways. Understanding this is very useful.

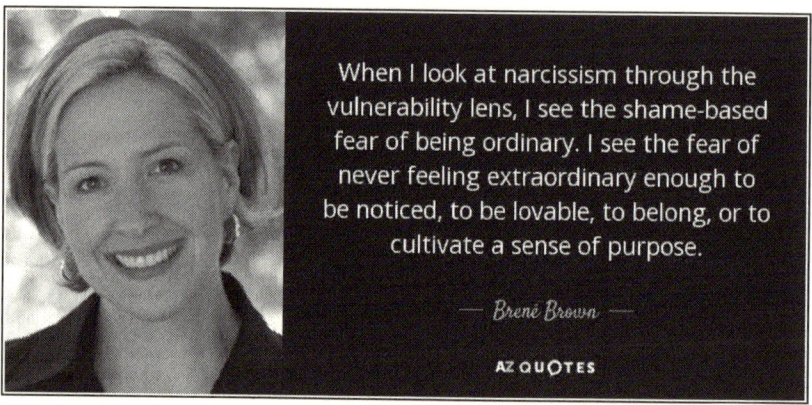

A very interesting study presented at **Psychology Today** suggests some socio-economic factors affect narcissism. The findings of the in-depth research suggest that people with very wealthy parents have a much higher level of self-importance. This sense of entitlement can lead to someone being more susceptible to narcissistic traits. While this isn't always the case, it's very interesting to consider and it might relate to your current situation.

4 Little-Known Causes of Narcissism

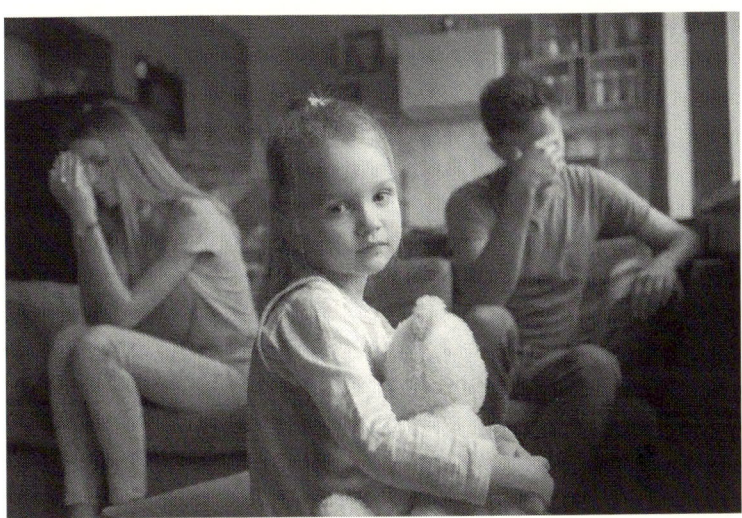

So, where does this shame come from? What causes it to manifest itself in such a way in people? Elinor Greenberg, PhD (study at *psychologytoday.com/blog/understanding-narcissism/201705/how-do-children-become-narcissists*) believes that it is all down to parenting, that your youth affects you in ways you didn't think possible when you're an adult. She gives **four examples of parenting styles that can lead to narcissism later:**

- *Love is conditional*

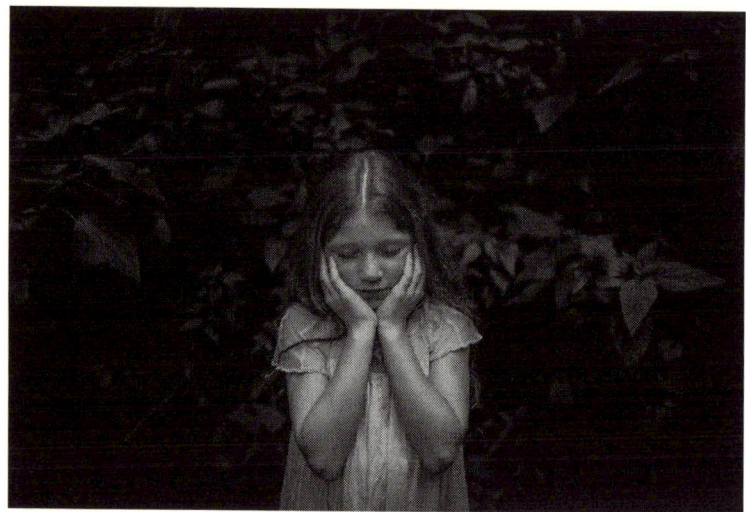

Children who are showered with praise when they achieve something but ignored the rest of the time can grow up feeling like the pressure is never off. They need people to understand how important they are because it's the only way they can get attention and affection. The pressure they can put on themselves to always succeed can be crushing inside.

If this is the case, then you need to ensure that the other person knows that they are unconditionally loved by you. That doesn't mean give and give without getting anything in return; it might just take a healthy, calm conversation to ensure the message is received.

- *The defeated child*

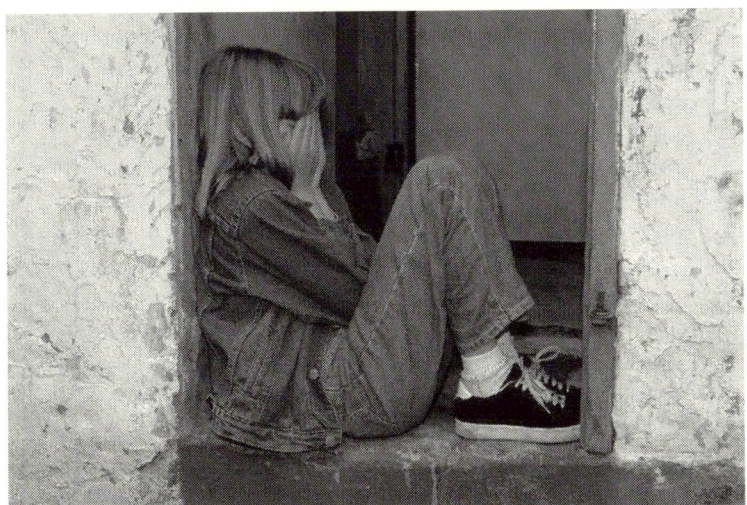

This person has grown up in a home with high expectations and little ability to achieve them. The parents were easily angered, highly irritable, and fostered feelings of inadequacy. This might come in the form of valuing one child so much more than another. It's a toxic and unhealthy upbringing that leads to an equally terrible adulthood with the need to prove themselves and get out their anger in various ways.

Someone who has suffered this will need to speak to a licensed therapist to overcome those emotions. A person who believes themselves to be truly unlovable can then not really love someone else, which creates a vicious cycle. Their loved ones will need to help with this time of change, with patience and love, *if* the narcissist is willing to put in the work.

- *The golden child*

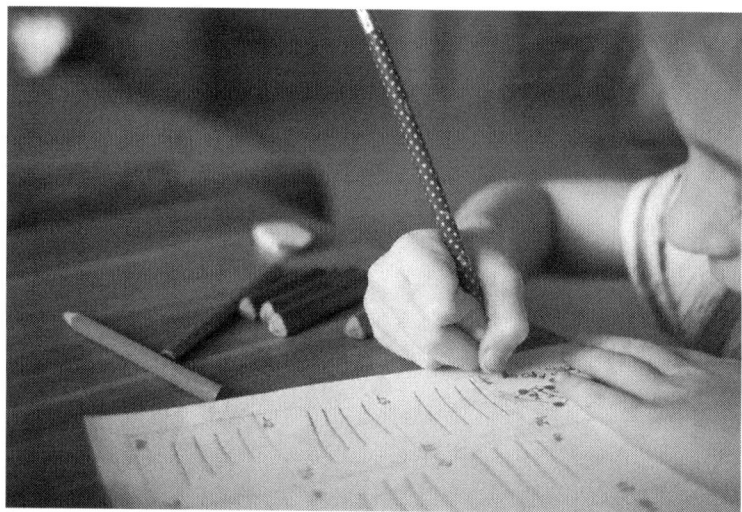

This child usually comes from parents who are closet narcissists but are uncomfortable with the spotlight, so they use their child's achievements as a way to gain indirect attention. The child may deserve this attention, but it's taken to an extreme level, leaving the child with narcissistic and perfectionist tendencies in later life.

To help someone who has suffered this, you need to help them see that weakness isn't a flaw and that no one can be perfect at everything. This is something that we will examine throughout this book.

- *Admiring the narcissist*

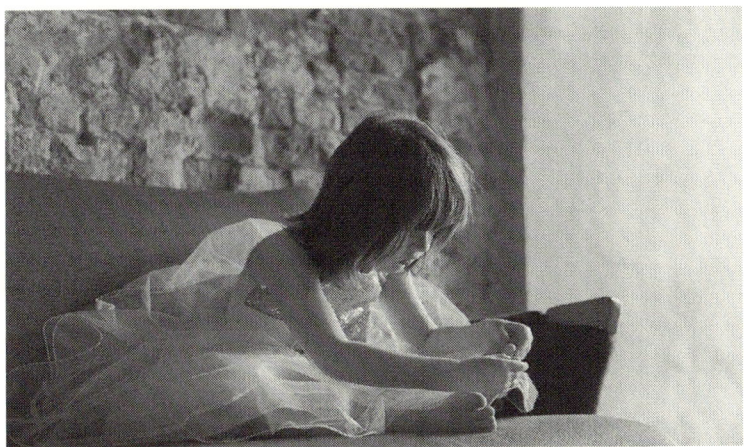

The narcissistic parent who discourages that sort of behavior in their child by refusing to compliment them encourages a competitive element within them. By the time adulthood comes around, their narcissistic might be less obvious but they *will* display symptoms of low self-esteem, yet they'll put themselves first.

This is another area of narcissism that requires the help of a trained professional, as the issues will be deep-rooted and need to be examined.

This can be seen in the case study presented by Jonice Webb, PhD (at blogs.psychcentral.com/childhood-neglect/2015/07/a-surprising-cause-of-narcissism), who suggests neglect creates negative emotions that continue on into later life, using the example of two different children who have had very different experiences, but have a similar outlook later on in life:

No one noticed when 8-year-old Bill came home sad and afraid from being bullied at school. He knew that he had to handle it himself, so he did.

No one noticed when Marcy was bullied either. But when she came home sad and afraid, her mother sent her to her room until she could "stop sulking."

Child Bill was overlooked at his large family's annual reunions.

At Child Marcy's family reunions, she was displayed by her parents for the relatives to admire her beauty; then she was essentially pushed to the side and ignored. At one reunion, teen Marcy refused to put on makeup. She wore old jeans and a ripped t-shirt. Her parents were so enraged at her refusal make them proud that they totally ignored her at the reunion and refused to acknowledge her existence for weeks after.

Bill's childhood taught him that his feelings and needs didn't matter. So he pushed them down, and lost access to his own emotions. He is living his adult life without a major source of connection, stimulation, and information. This is the "flaw" which he senses deeply, but has no words to describe.

Marcy lives her life in the grip of a terrible fear; a fear of being unnoticed. "Look at me! Look at me! Look at me!", she calls out with her every word and her every act, "I matter! I matter! I matter!" Marcy only feels okay when she is in the limelight. She learned early and well that when she is not under a spotlight, she is nothing.

Yes, Bill and Marcy are very, very different. But deep down, they share this common core: I am empty. I am alone. I don't matter. I can't let others see me too closely. Because then they will see that I am nothing.

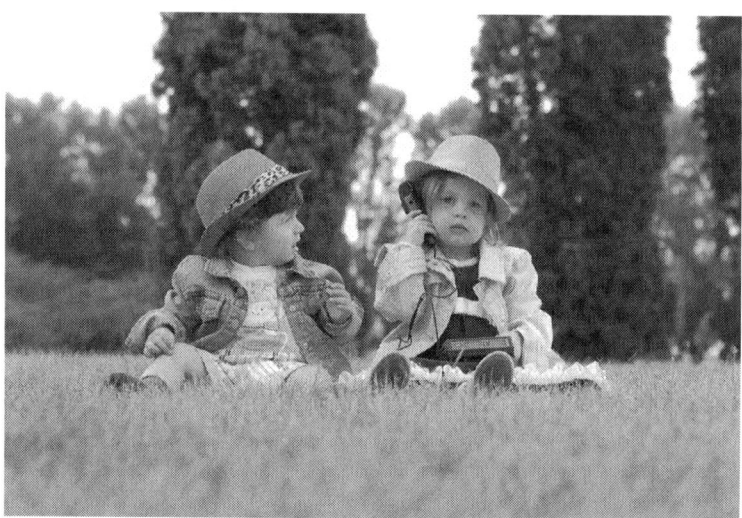

If this is something that you might fear for your child, and **you wish to combat the issue early on,** here are some tips:

- Teach empathy.
- Place value on traits like kindness and honesty more than being dominant or tough.
- Change entitled attitudes and stop entitled actions.
- Squelch greed (say, "You're acting selfishly and that's not okay").
- Insist they put other people first routinely, remembering that actions speak louder than words (narcissists often say they are doing something to benefit others when they are really doing it for themselves).
- Build healthy self-esteem (low self-esteem can also lead to entitlement and using others to support one's ego).
- Don't allow false blame of other people for one's own problems and failures.
- Avoid parenting styles linked to developing a narcissistic personality, such as neglecting, indulgent (spoiling with privilege and possessions, and promoting entitled attitudes), and controlling and cold authoritari-

an methods that focus on toughness, winning, and perfection from a child.
- Help teens and young adults learn to recognize narcissists so they can avoid their toxic harm or survive it.

> ### Narcissistic Parents
> "Children of selfish and demanding parents are not guilty of anything. They have been abused and manipulated into believing that their sole purpose is to make their parent happy. In fact, this is a destructive con job, and the guilt rests with the self-absorbed or narcissistic parent."
>
> — Glynis Sherwood, MEd

The Science of Narcissism

A lot of scientific research has been published exploring narcissism, and because of that, we can see the difference in brain activity. A study conducted by Dr. Syras Derksen (at *drsyrasderksen.com/seeing-narcissism-in-the-brain.html*) has revealed many interesting things. The main discovery is that the empathy part of the brain is much less developed, which explains a lot of the behavior associated with the disorder.

The report of this study, which employed MRI scans of normal and narcissistic brains, showed that:

"People with this disorder can take the perspective of another person in a purely intellectual way. However, when it comes to actually feeling what another person is going through, narcissists have difficulty."

This means that narcissists understand the emotions of others in a very different, more clinical way than everyone else. So, despite the fact that this sort of behavior is learned throughout life, it does have a profound effect on the brain. All hope isn't lost, though, because with some work, these effects *can* be reversed.

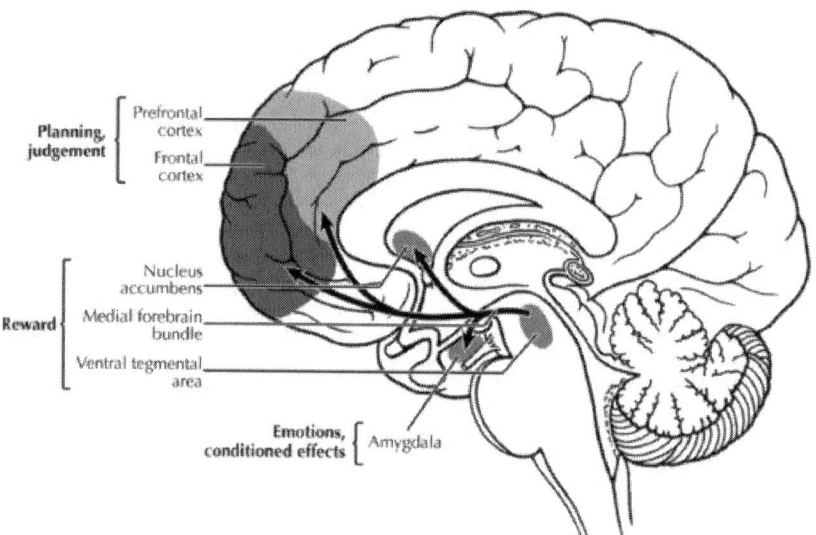

Another study, presented at *Live Science* (at *www.livescience.com/37684-narcissistic-personality-disorder-brain-structure.html*), confirms this. The research conducted compared brain scans of 34 people, 17 with narcissistic personality disorder, and they found that the suffers of the disorder have much less gray matter in the cerebral cortex of the brain. This area of the brain is involved with cognitive functioning and the regulation of emotion. So, without it, sufferers are less able to deal with their own emotions, much less those of others.

"Our data shows that the amount of empathy is directly correlated to the volume of gray brain matter of the corresponding cortical representation in the insular region, and that the patients with narcissism exhibit a structural deficit in exactly this area," states Dr. Röpke, commenting on the findings. *"Building on this initial structural data, we are currently attempting to use functional imaging (fMRI) to understand better how the brains of patients with narcissistic personality disorder work."*

There is still a lot of work to go before scientists can fully understand this condition, but work is always being done, as shown at the *Harvard Scientist Review* (at *harvardsciencereview.com/2015/12/03/the-simple-science-of-a-grandiose-mind*). The closer scientists and doctors get to learning everything about it, the better the treatment programs will become.

60-Second Narcissism Quiz

ARE YOU A NARCISSIST?

Check the following list of common narcissistic personality traits and see how many you relate to:

SELF-CENTERED
- ✓ Constantly thinking about yourself
- ✓ Focus on getting your own needs met (often ignoring the needs of others)

SENSE OF ENTITLEMENT OR SUPERIORITY
- ✓ Feeling that you are always right
- ✓ Feeling that you are better or deserve more than other people

LACK OF EMPATHY
- ✓ Lacking compassion and feeling for other people

MANIPULATIVE OR CONTROLLING
- ✓ Use emotions to manipulate people
- ✓ Tendency to be extremely jealous and controlling in relationships

STRONG NEED FOR ADMIRATION
- ✓ Demand admiration and praise
- ✓ Like to be the center of attention
- ✓ Upset if the spotlight is not on you

DIFFICULTY TAKING FEEDBACK
- ✓ Over-react to criticism
- ✓ Have a hard time admitting when you are wrong

EASILY WOUNDED
- ✓ Quick to feel hurt or angry
- ✓ Frequently feel wronged by others

Here is a quiz designed **to see if someone you know is a narcissist**. This can also apply to you, if you suspect this might be something you're suffering from. If that's the case, simply rephrase the questions to apply to you.

- If something bad happens, will they blame others first?
- Have they often refused to accept responsibility for bad behavior?
- Do they act as if they are always right?
- Do they struggle understanding others' feelings?
- Do they show more concern for how others' behavior will affect them?
- Are they denying their feelings, then getting defensive about it?
- Are they prone to holding grudges?
- Do they focus on their demands and wishes?
- Are they unwilling to hear you out or listen to you?
- Do they always tell people what to do?
- Are they living in the belief other people are never good enough?
- Will they avoid asking how other people are doing?
- Are they reminding you of their greatness regularly, even when it's a lie or an exaggeration of the truth?
- Are they often telling lies?
- Are they manipulative?
- Will they manipulate or spin the truth so they end up looking good?
- When they include people they know in conversation, is it so they can boast?
- Have you noticed that others hesitate in spending time with them?
- Are others not willing to share ideas and feelings around them?
- Are they mistrustful of people?
- Do people in their life have to work to gain their approval and love?
- Are they spending a minimal amount of time with their child or children?
- Will they typically choose to skip events if they see no personal value in it?
- Do other people mention that something is strange or different about them?
- Will they use other people for personal gain?

- Do they focus on control and power, seeking power by any means?
- Do they obsess over image and making things look good to others?
- Do they act like they have no clear value system, no concrete opinion of right and wrong?
- Are they always turning the subject of a conversation back to themselves?
- Are they always trying to top others' stories with their own?
- Are they often jealous of people they know?
- Are they lacking in empathy?
- Are they only supportive of things that will make them look good?
- Have others mentioned feeling a lack of emotional connection from them?
- Are they only doing good so people can witness it?
- Do they show no concern when something difficult happens to others?
- Do they spend a lot of time worrying what others will think?
- Have they taken advantage of others who have been kind in the past?
- Have they made people feel responsible for their sicknesses or ailments?
- Do they struggle with accepting other people?
- Are they easily condescending and judgmental toward people?
- Do they refuse to take the time to try to get to know people better?
- Are they acting in the belief the world revolves around them and their needs?
- Do they come off as fake or a fraud to you or others?
- Does their mood swing from depression to grandiosity?
- Are they always acting like they have to compete with people?
- Are they inflexible with how other people get things done?

If the answer to these questions was more 'yes' than 'no,' then this book is definitely for you. You need to read on to work out how to end this vicious narcissistic cycle you're in. As previously stated, things can be done to improve your situation, so don't lose hope.

When Does This Become a *Real* Issue?

Narcissistic tendencies are always problematic, but there are times when it is worse than others. A 'healthy' dose of narcissism can actually be beneficial to you. This is defined as having self-esteem, while still maintaining a connection to others. It is self-love without being detrimental to others.

Characteristic	Healthy Narcissism
Self-confidence	High outward self-confidence in line with reality
Desire for power, wealth and admiration	May enjoy power
Relationships	Real concern for others and their ideas; does not exploit or devalue others
Ability to follow a consistent path	Has values; follows through on plans
Foundation	Healthy childhood with support for self-esteem and appropriate limits on behavior towards others

In fact, it's seen as so beneficial that we even have **some tips to help you gain some narcissism in your life to boost confidence** when times are tough:

- Focus on how you feel on the inside, not how you look on the outside.
- Establish your own identity; don't worry what others expect of you.
- Feel proud when you reach your goals.
- Set out to achieve your aims and accept your strengths and weaknesses.
- Give yourself affirmations.
- Consider what you like about yourself.
- Care for yourself.
- Be kind to yourself, but also to others.
- Allow yourself to have imperfections.
- Encourage and allow yourself to have a wide range of feelings.
- When you feel bad, do something to change it.
- Share in the success of others.

However, this isn't always the case. Sometimes the **narcissistic tendencies are extreme** and need some serious changes to be made. If this is something you fear might be affecting you or someone in your life, please read on for more information.

1. Sociopath

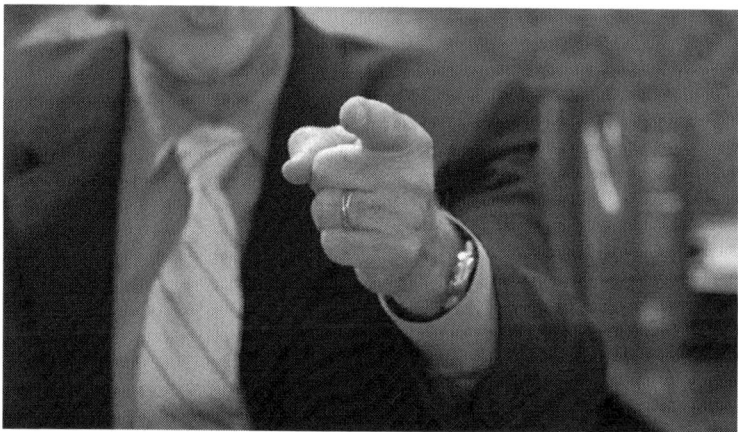

A sociopath is someone who is usually defined by lack of empathy. Someone with an antisocial personality is often seen as a sociopath as they do not interact with others in the way that people without this form of narcissism do. They're known for being very charming and likable, but this is all a façade. Underneath all of that superficial falseness, they're calculating and have controlling behavior.

Here is **a list of symptoms to look out for**:

- Being deceitful and lying. For example, they might con others and feel no remorse or use an alias to hide themselves or what they're doing.
- An inability to follow social norms. They may act in inappropriate ways, from speaking out of turn to breaking the law.
- Overly assertive or aggressive behavior. They may be prone to getting into physical fights.
- An absence of empathy for others' feelings, even if they are responsible for those feelings.
- A display of very shallow feelings.
- Impulsive behavior that can hinder planning for the future.
- Lack of concern for others' safety.
- Irresponsibility that drives inconsistent behavior.

- Taking part in reckless behavior, such as stealing, promiscuity, and taking uncalculated risks.

This behavior is worrying because it can lead to abusive relationships, aggression, and even violence. The longer that people allow it to continue, the worse it will get. The further a sociopath will push the boundaries to see what they can get away with. It needs to be dealt with immediately to protect everyone who comes into contact with this person.

If you know someone who shows no remorse for their actions, no matter what they've done, and they also don't recognize that they have something they need to change about themselves, then they might be a narcissistic sociopath. Studies have shown this also often emanates from neglecting parents, sociopathic parents, or traumatic, abusive events. This can best be treated with the help of a medical professional, and it's usually done via therapy.

2. Psychopath

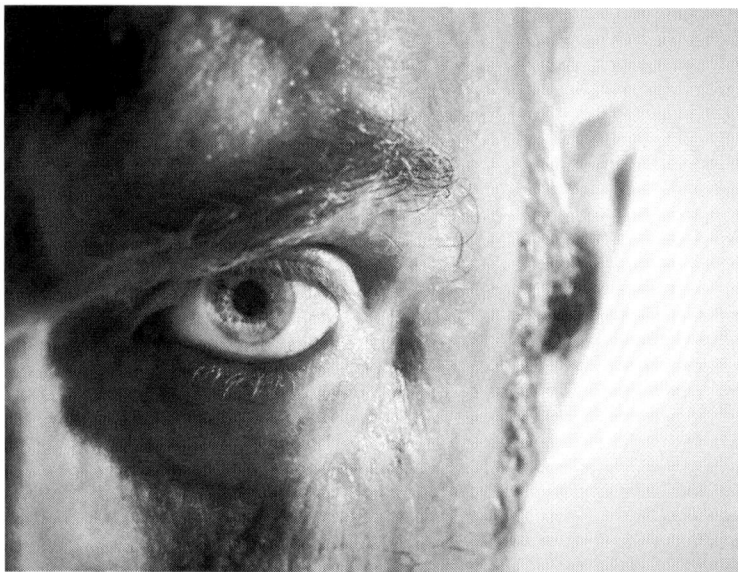

Joshua Buckholtz, an associate professor of psychology at Harvard, conducted a study with prisoners to learn more about their tendency towards poor decision-making and violence. What was found is *"psychopaths' brains are wired in a way that leads them to over-value immediate rewards and neglect the future consequences of potentially dangerous or immoral actions."*

Before this study, it has always been believed that psychopaths lack emotions and empathy, but it's more that they don't consider what will happen next. This makes sense when you think about the amount of criminals who display these tendencies, but another research project found that fully functioning, successful adults with high-flying careers also show the same brain activity as a psychopath.

Here are **some ways you can detect a psychopath**:

- Superficial charm to lure people in at first.
- Ignoring huge problems with a non-committal attitude.
- An inflated sense of self.
- A need for stimulation from extreme activities.
- Lying, conning, manipulating.
- Lack of guilt even when pain is caused.
- Shallow feelings, no depth of emotions.
- No empathy.

- Poor control, promiscuous behavior, other behavioral issues.
- Impulsive, irresponsible, no long-term goals.
- A tendency towards criminal activity.

The earlier these tendencies are spotted, the more chance you have at helping someone. By allowing this behavior to continue, you are letting it get worse. Psychopaths will use your weaknesses against you to get what they want. The best thing you can do for yourself is to extract yourself from the situation if possible, before you get harmed. If doing this really isn't possible, then you need some medical help for your loved one.

3. Narcopath

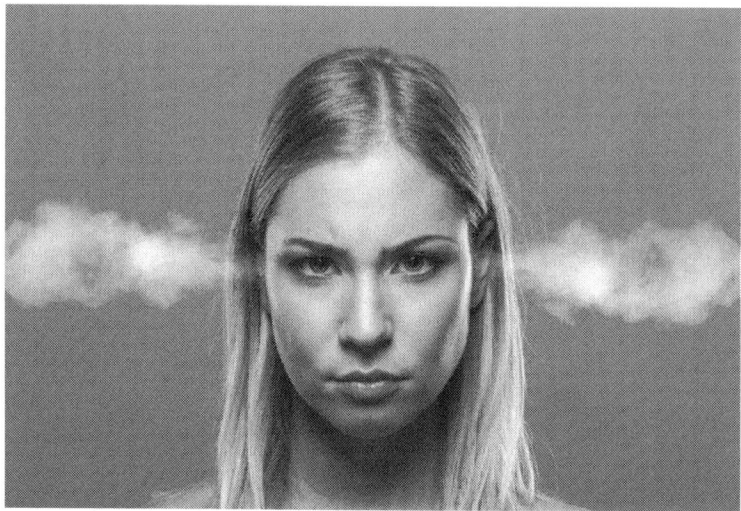

A narcopath is a narcissist-sociopath mix and is considered the worst type. Someone with an inflated sense of how important they are, as well as a constant need for praise and admiration – which already sounds exhausting! Relationships with them can be addictive, but draining as the person with a narcopath will never win.

Here is **a great checklist for identifying whether you are involved with a narcopath**:

- Things move fast – really fast! Instead of spending time getting to know you, a narcopath will immediately make you feel like you've found your soul mate.
- The compliments – at first, they might feel nice, but after a while, you might realize that they're generic and may be a bit staged.
- Flattery comes in the form of comparisons. This is especially bad if it links to an ex. Even if you come out on top, that won't last.
- You have a strong chemistry. The passion is off the charts, but not much else is good.
- Hollow eyes that lead to nothing. It's all an act.
- The conversation always swivels back to themselves.
- A checkered relationship history is a sign of things to come.
- The silent treatment is common.

This is another serious form of narcissism that can lead to abuse and violence if left untreated. It isn't always easy to confront someone who behaves in such a way, but doing so can lead to a happier future for the perpetrator and everyone in their life. Some therapy, especially cognitive behavioral therapy, can help with this.

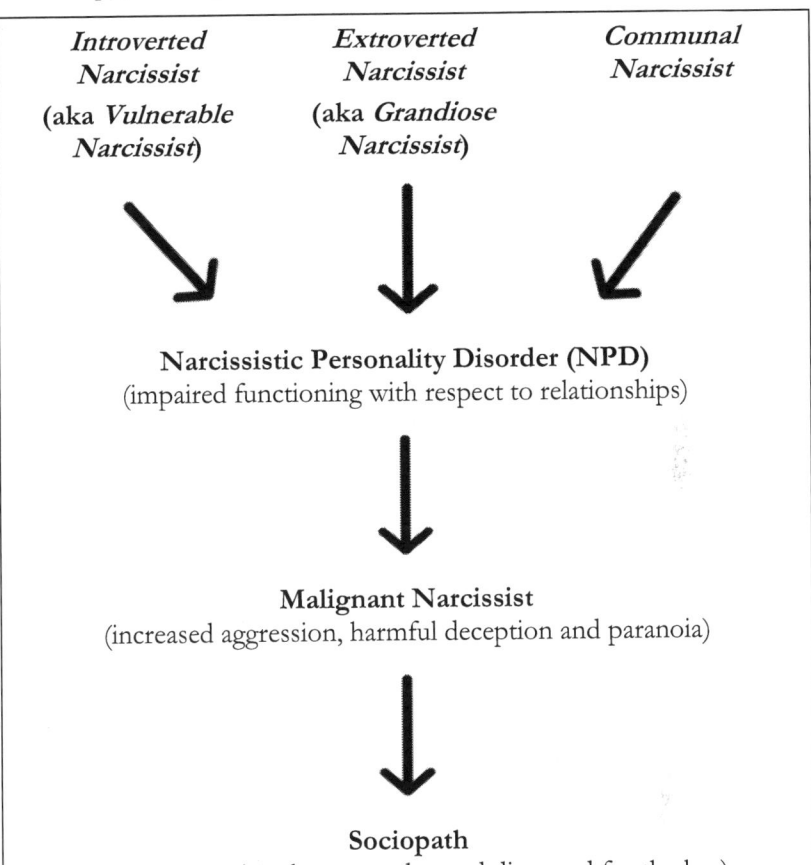

The red flags of manipulation include:
- Your words being used against you.
- They offer you help, but their help leaves you confused and unhappy.
- They say shocking things, then claim that you misunderstood them.
- A lot of what they do is designed to make you feel guilt and shame.
- You question your own sanity.
- Love and affection are withdrawn once you don't obey them.
- You fear losing that person, no matter what they do.
- You always feel like you fall short of expectations.
- You have to walk on eggshells around that person.
- You feel isolated by them.

If you feel any of these things happening in your life, then you need to start thinking about taking some serious action. Read on for ways to help yourself and the narcissism sufferer.

8 Surprising Narcissism Facts

	SELF LOVE		NARCISSISM
✓	Healthy self-esteem	✗	False sense of high self-esteem
✓	Respects free will of self and others	✗	Likes to control others
✓	Happy & fulfilled	✗	Nothing is ever good enough
✓	Humble	✗	Grandiose
✓	Enjoys time alone	✗	Always needs people around
✓	Free of other's opinions	✗	Very concerned with what others think
✓	Self-assured	✗	Outwardly charming but deeply insecure
✓	Empathic towards others	✗	Manipulative & callous of others
✓	Empowering of others	✗	Degrading of others

You might think that you know everything about narcissism, or at least a lot more by now, but here are some facts that might just shock you into rethinking and opening your mind a little to just who might be affected by this disorder:

1. A study has shown that wealth is the biggest socio-economic factor affecting narcissism. More money can lead to a greater sense of entitlement (*psychologytoday.com/blog/ulterior-motives/201401/rich-entitled-and-narcissistic*).
2. A research project discovered that it's mostly men who suffer from narcissistic tendencies (*healthresearchfunding.org/odd-narcissistic-personality-disorder-statistics*).
3. 17% of narcissists actually fall under the 'extreme' type listed above.
4. *Barends Psychology* has found that narcissism tends to be more prevalent among African Americans (12.5%) when compared to the Hispanic (7.5%) and Caucasian (5.0%) populations (*barendspsychology.com/narcissism-facts*).
5. The term 'narcissism' was borrowed by Freud, who examined it closely, from Paul Näcke, who, in 1899, explored a type of behavior, almost a perversion, where an individual would treat their body in the same way they might treat the body of a romantic partner.
6. According to Jeffrey Kluger, social media isn't to blame for our narcissism; it's just a great place for us to display it for the world to see (*mprnews.org/story/2014/10/23/daily-circuit-jeffrey-kluger*).
7. 6.2% of the people have narcissism. 7.7% of the men and 4.8% of the women.

NARCISSISTIC PERSONALITY DISORDER FACTS

6.2% of people has narcissism once in their lives

7.7% **4.8%**

7.7% OF MEN DEVELOP NARCISSISM COMPARED TO 4.8% OF WOMEN

DISABILITY IS ASSOCIATED WITH NARCISSISM AMONG MEN, BUT NOT AMONG WOMEN

MEN WITH NARCISSISM HAVE HIGHER RATES OF MOST SUBSTANCE ABUSE DISORDERS AND ANTISOCIAL PERSONALITY DISORDER

WOMEN WITH NARCISSISM HAVE HIGHER RATES OF MAJOR DEPRESSIVE DISORDER AND MOST ANXIETY DISORDERS

- **82.1%** THINKS THEY ARE UNIQUE OR SPECIAL
- **80.4%** HAS A SENSE OF ENTITLEMENT
- **78.8%** SHOWS LACK OF EMPATHY

UNMARRIED, SEPARATED, DIVORCED AND WIDOWED PEOPLE MORE OFTEN HAVE NARCISSISM

NARCISSISM IS MORE COMMON AMONG ADULTS AGED 20-29 (9.4%) COMPARED TO ADULTS AGED 30-44 (7.1%) AND 45-64 (5.6%)

ETHNICITY:

- AFRO-AMERICANS: 12.5%
- HISPANICS: 7.5%
- NATIVE AMERICAN: 7.1%
- ASIAN / PACIFIC : 5.4%
- CAUCASIANS: 5.0%

WWW.BARENDSPSYCHOLOGY.COM

8. There is a very strong belief that narcissism cannot be overcome. This book is going to show you that isn't the case at all.

14 Narcissism Facts...and the tips that don't love them back

N-**Nothing** you say, do or promise will get them to change. Change is as foreign, feared and toxic as cancer is to the rest of humanity.

A-**Always** watch your back because she'll strike when you least expect it.

R-**Reach out** to a qualified mental health professional when the rage causes you to wonder, *"Am I going crazy?"*

C-**Children** have one shot at childhood. Protect them from physical harm and emotional abuse. Same goes for pets, and other vulnerable populations.

I-**"I" statements** such as "I feel like you're not listening" can help you assert your wants and needs. Even if the civility falls on deaf ears.

S-**Studies show** men who possess traits of entitlement and exploitation show elevated levels of cortisol, a stress hormone linked to high blood pressure and heart problems.

S-**Some narcissistic females** rate high for histrionic traits (obsessively craving attention, drama and sexual approval, etc). She may be hot, but run for the hills when she hits you up at work, the party, the club and Starbucks.

I-**"Imaginary audiences** that follow them everywhere," is one faulty belief causing teens to think everyone is impressed by their behaviors. The god news is most people mature as they develop interpersonal relationships, responsibilities and raise families.

S-**Stand up** to the bullying and learn to impose firm boundaries.

M-**Marriage?** Say it ain't so. Trust me. I know.

T-**Throw in the towel** if you don't like competition. **Team N** believes in The Winners vs The Losers. And you, my friend are a perennial pawn on the losing team.

I-**Involve** yourself with a support group if you're married to The Egomaniac.

P-**Practice** deep-breathing, relaxation, and walking away. Keep going until you reach the intersection of **Better Than This** and **Sanity**.

S-**Survival** depends on these strategies and more, in order to preserve your precious mental health. *You deserve better.*

by Linda Esposito, LCSW
www.talktherapybiz.com

25 PROVEN STEPS TO DISCOVER NARCISSISM

An Ideal Target

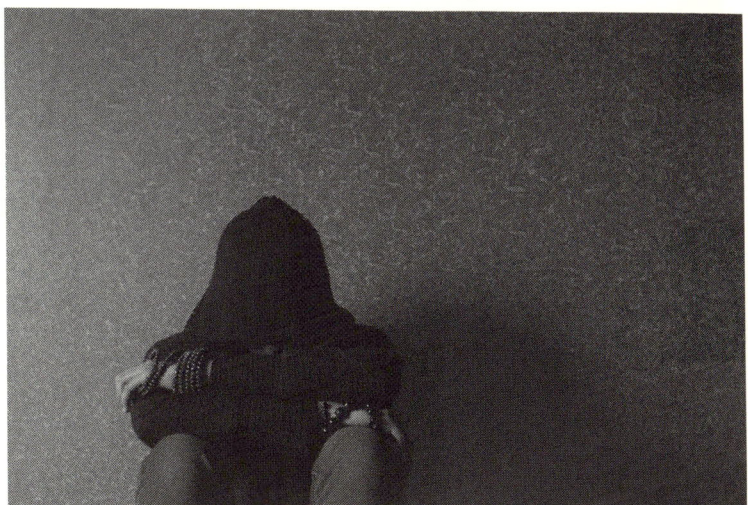

If you have been targeted by a narcissist, you might be wondering *why*. What attracted them to you? What made you their victim? Well, some **research has been done into this and here are the results**:

1. Narcissists choose empathetic, compassionate people. Basically the opposite to them!
2. It can also be someone who will feed their ego. Someone with a low self-esteem of their own. Someone they can manipulate into living life their way.
3. Someone with something that others will envy – money, power, beau-

ty, anything to add value to themselves.
4. They may also choose someone who they know loves them more than themselves. This makes them much more likely to accept blame than anyone else.
5. A 'challenge.' A strong, confident partner that they can knock down. Narcissists often don't enjoy life and don't want others to either.

What a Narcissist Wants?

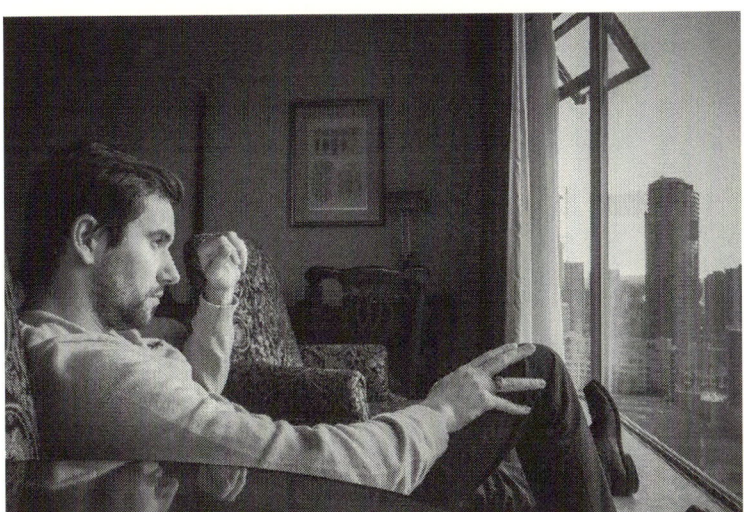

What does the narcissist in your life want from you? Well, this can be a number of things. It's up to you to **determine which item from the list most suits your situation**:

1. They want to spread their feelings of misery, failure, and rejection around so it doesn't only feel like it's happening to them.
2. Drama. The narcissist often gets bored very quickly, so they will do anything they can to make everything very dramatic and exciting. It can feel like a terrifying roller-coaster.
3. A narcissistic supply. Someone to feed their constant need for attention.
4. A one-way-street relationship, which leaves them with all the power.
5. Someone who will accept the mask and never delve around to what's underneath, where all the fear and shame is hidden.

The Effect on Me

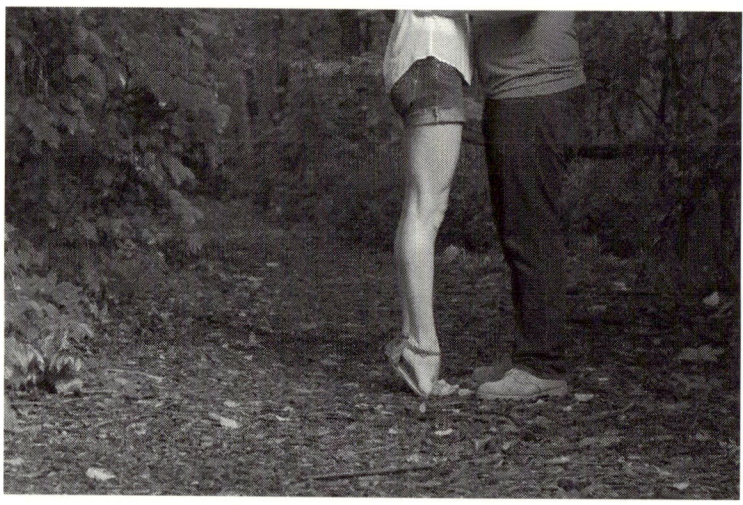

How does this behavior affect you? What impact will it have on the lives of everyone around them? Often, the narcissist person isn't affected by their own behavior at all, which means **they don't see it as the issue everyone else does**:

1. When a narcissist denies something so much, and so confidently, it can leave the other person wondering if they are in the wrong, doubting what they have previously believed and maybe even questioning their own sanity. Denial and self-doubt become a very vicious cycle.
2. It can feel phenomenal when everything is going well and the narcissist is happy. This feeling is like a drug and has people coming back for more. It's dizzying, thrilling, passionate. Often, you're still chasing this high, even when it doesn't come around anymore.
3. The crushing lows when nothing is going to *their* plan are hard to deal with. You're constantly treading on eggshells trying to prevent this from happening. The constant sense that drama could come your way leaves you jittery and without any self-confidence.
4. Your own happiness is *much* less important. You might even stop thinking of yourself at all...
5. ...which leads to you blaming yourself for things that you haven't done, or at least accepting the blame for an easy life.

6 Secret Tools Narcissists Use for Emotional Manipulation

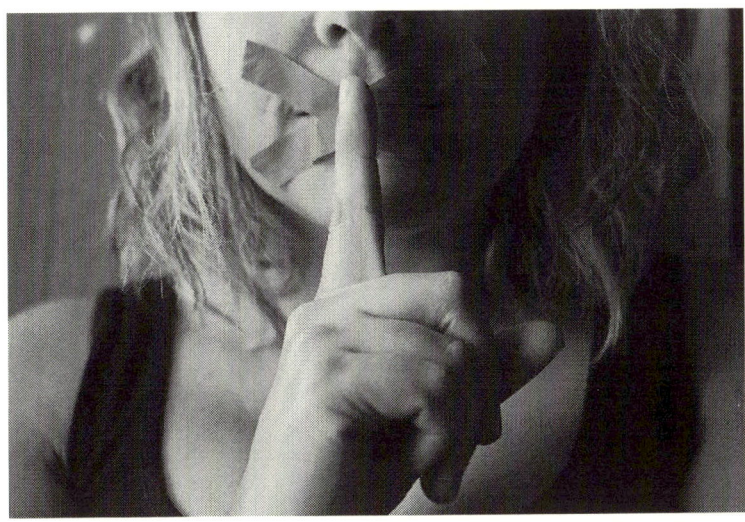

Narcissists will use emotional manipulation to ensure they get what they want. It can start with charm and happiness, but once it gets past that part, they need **new tactics to ensure everything is as they want it**. Some of these can include:

1. When they're challenged, the narcissist can use mostly nonsensical monologues to distract from the real issue, to the point where it's impossible to even talk to them.
2. Moving the goalpost so you can never please them. If the victim is a people pleaser, this is a great tactic to keep them feeding the narcissist's ego.
3. Name-calling, blaming others, changing the subject – anything to take the conversation in another direction.
4. Shaming, which might come in the form of condescension, patronization, or jokes at your expense – anything to make them feel like they have the upper hand against you. They want to make sure that you know it too.
5. Deflecting and acting like they are the victim, to the point where you wonder if it might actually be the truth!

The tools that narcissists use to inflict this emotional abuse to trick their victim into feeling inferior and causing them to feel trapped in their cycle can include:

- *Enmeshment* – this is a concept introduced by Salvador Minuchin to describe families or couples in which the personal boundaries are unclear. The emotions of one person will impact on the whole house, they will be 'felt' by everyone, but in a very toxic way. This leaves the victim tiptoeing on eggshells, unsure of how they are allowed to feel and behave themselves. In this case, when things are good, they are amazing, which traps the victim into thinking that the bad times aren't all that bad.

- *Psychological Love Starvation* – having love deprived and making the victim feel desperate for it is not real love, it's emotional abuse. If you find yourself insecure of the narcissist's love, then their trap is working. This is how they keep you wanting to stay, because you constantly feel like you need to fight for them.

- *Guilt* – this is a narcissist's favorite tool because it's very easy to feel it. It's there inside of us always, and it's simple to ignite. They will make you feel like everything is your fault and that you should behave in a certain way because of the sacrifices that they have made for you. This is all about control, and it's hard to break free from, but recognizing it is an important first step.

- *Low Shame Tolerance* – shame is a driving force for narcissism. They already feel a lot of shame for things that have happened in their past, so any new shame, even if it isn't related to them, creates panic within them. They will turn everything around to keep the attention only on them no matter what happens. Eventually, the victim will inadvertently think that the world revolves around the narcissist.

- *Fear* – the victim will eventually become trapped in a cycle of fear. They will become so afraid of hurting or 'setting off' the narcissist that escape won't even feel like an option anymore.

- *Shamelessness* – while narcissists suffer from shame, they also are shameless when it comes to certain behaviors. Because they live a life without limits, sometimes they forget about reality and norms. When they aim to get what they want, they are shameless on who they trample over along the way. This makes them terrible friends, lovers, and parents because they think only of themselves.

5 Subtle Signs to Look Out For

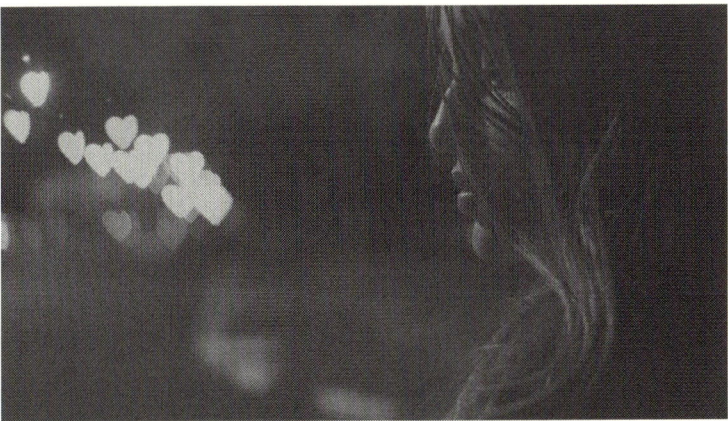

Red flags of narcissistic behavior start early on in a relationship, and if you're wiser to them, you'll be able to spot them better.

1. There are three stages of a narcissistic relationship. ***Idealization***, where they will become full-on romantic to catch you. ***Devaluation***, where they will start to put their victim down in a way that makes the victim feel dependent on them. ***Discard*** is the final stage, and it's done in the most public, humiliating way possible, often via cheating.
2. ***Gaslighting*** is another thing that narcissistic people are known to do, so the victim doesn't see the perspective of blame for where it really is. They blame themselves.
3. Someone who changes who they are depending on who they're with is something to be concerned about. It means there is a constant mask in the way, and it's impossible to tell who the real person is.
4. Creating an environment of instability and self-doubt helps narcissists greatly. By feeding into worries of the relationship being stripped away, ensures that you're always competing for their attention, feeding their ego along the way.
5. Pushing your boundaries, even on little things to see how far they can get around you. This will be littered with over-the-top apologies when you react, but the behavior is a pattern that will come around again.

All of this behavior is troubling, and once you recognize it, you will need to change it before you can move forward. It's vital that you do not stay in the situation as it is because it will not get better. The good news is that things *can* be fixed. It isn't a hopeless situation with no solution. It just takes some input from both sides.

The next few chapters will help you to start this journey.

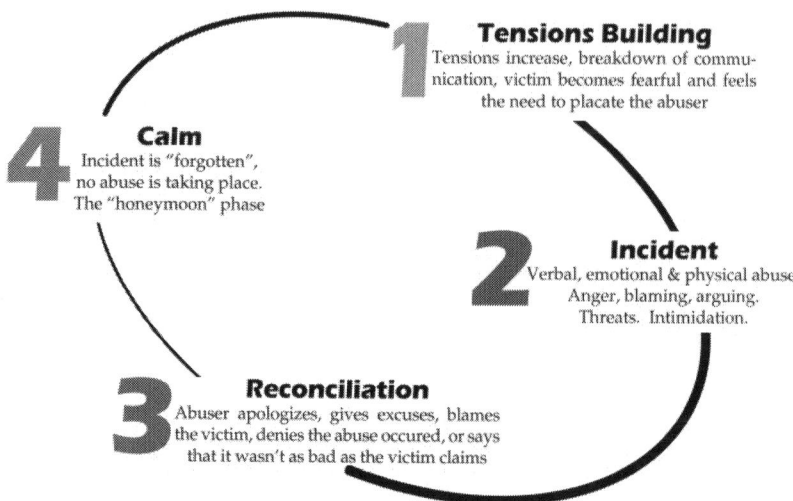

10 UNEXPLORED WAYS NARCISSISM AFFECTS YOU

When you are living with a narcissist, it can affect many different areas of your existence, even in ways you didn't expect. This chapter gives you some insight into how deep this goes so you can unpack where *you* are being affected. Identifying this is the first step towards recovering from it.

1. Your Life

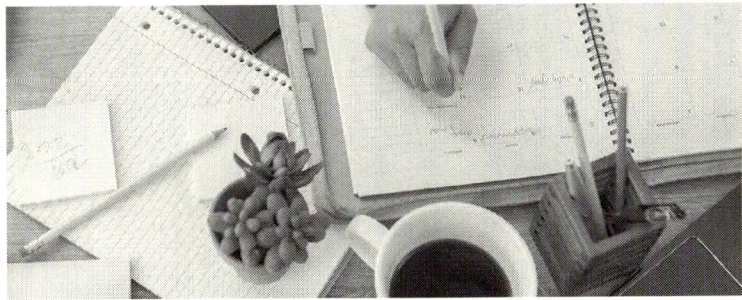

Living in a narcissistic abusive relationship cycle can affect all the areas of your life. It's an issue from the moment you wake up to the moment you go to sleep, probably even affecting your dreams. It makes your home life uncomfortable, your time at work unpleasant, never mind spending time with other people. That can even become impossible.

Living with someone who only thinks of themselves and belittles everyone around them can have a very negative impact. If you're experiencing a lower self-esteem than you used to, then this might be something that you want to look into.

Preston Ni, M.S.B.A. has identified **the most common areas of life that are affected by narcissism.** For the victim and the perpetrator:

- *Family estrangement* – narcissism affects the wider circle of people as well, often causing rifts in previously very solid relationships.
- *Loneliness* – this can, of course, lead to feeling very alone, because no one really understands your situation and why you behave the way you do.
- *Missed opportunities* – with your social life, at work, you might not agree to do things that you would have before because you're afraid of the consequences.
- *Financial trouble* – narcissists will often put themselves first, and this can lead to money troubles as the bills and things that need to be paid might not come first.
- *Damaged reputation* – because you aren't acting like yourself, the way others view you may change, and not in a positive way.
- *Fear* – anxiety and images of rejection might start to consume you and leave you scared to leave the situation.

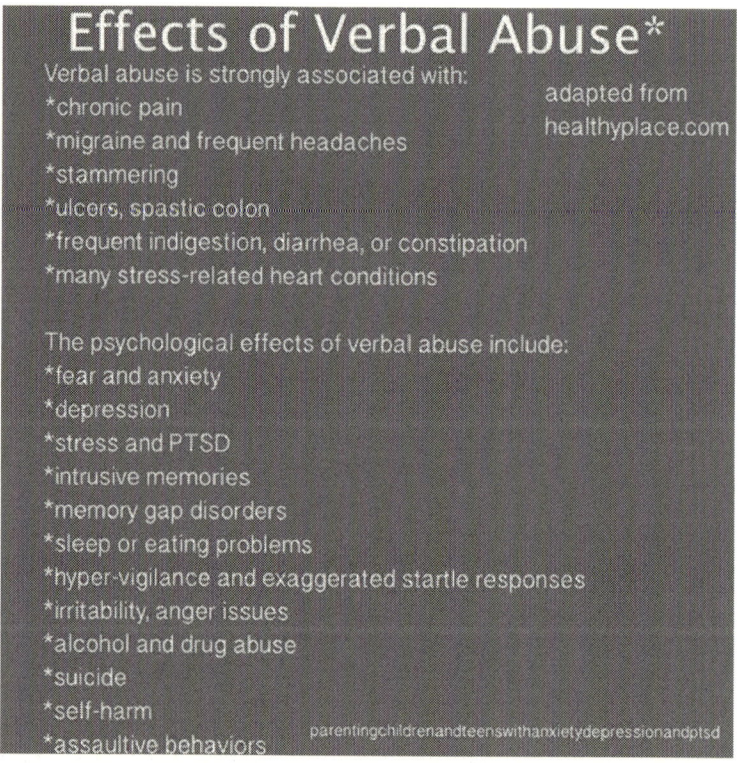

Effects of Verbal Abuse*

Verbal abuse is strongly associated with:
*chronic pain
*migraine and frequent headaches
*stammering
*ulcers, spastic colon
*frequent indigestion, diarrhea, or constipation
*many stress-related heart conditions

The psychological effects of verbal abuse include:
*fear and anxiety
*depression
*stress and PTSD
*intrusive memories
*memory gap disorders
*sleep or eating problems
*hyper-vigilance and exaggerated startle responses
*irritability, anger issues
*alcohol and drug abuse
*suicide
*self-harm
*assaultive behaviors

adapted from healthyplace.com

parentingchildrenandteenswithanxietydepressionandptsd

It can be difficult to extract yourself from a situation like this, that's left you dizzy and unsure of what's real. You've probably been told so many lies that it's difficult to differentiate. Then there's also the sensation of being foolish and knowing that everyone could see it but you. That doesn't make it impossible, though, as the following chapter of the book will help you to see.

2. Your Relationship

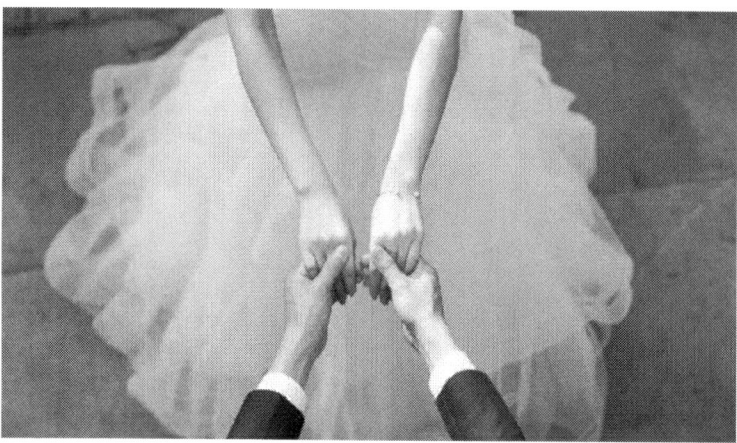

Living with someone who suffers from narcissism is never easy. Constantly being with someone who only thinks about themselves isn't easy for anyone and can bring your self-esteem right down. A study by the *Exhausted Woman* (at <u>pro.psychcentral.com/exhausted-woman/2015/05/the-narcissistic-cycle-of-abuse</u>) has shown **the four narcissistic cycles of abuse**. It doesn't necessarily work exactly as shown below, but if this is happening within your home, you should be able to recognize this in your life.

Read on to see if any of these apply to you:

- *Feeling threatened.* This happens to the narcissist. Something happens to make them feel threatened, and they become impossible to be around. This can be a minor rejection, an issue at work, some form of disapproval – anything. Then the person living with them is left terrified and walking on eggshells, while the narcissist obsesses over what happened at the expense of everyone else.

- *Abuse of others.* The abusive behavior will then begin. This might be making the spouse feel uncomfortable in their own home, nasty verbal comments, or something even worse. This will happen in such a way that the victim already feels locked in.

- *Becoming the victim.* Then, when the victim finally does something to stand up for themselves, the narcissist will flip things around and make the other person feel guilty. The narcissist will be very good at lying and turning things around so the victim will end up very confused.

- *Empowerment.* Once the victim feels like they are in the wrong, the narcissist is back in control. The more regularly the narcissist makes the victim feel like they are to blame, the easier it becomes for them to continue doing this. Then the cycle continues over and over again.

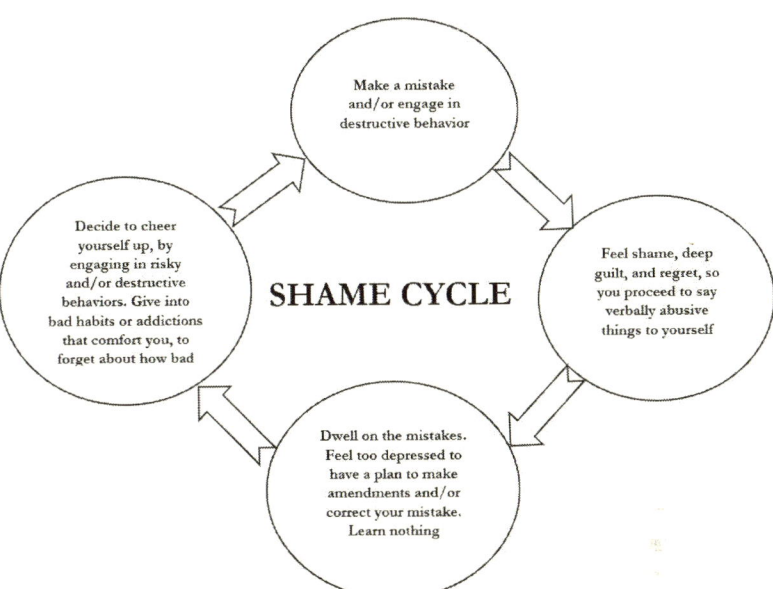

Shame is a big part of this cycle, as shown in a previous chapter. Shame is what the perpetrator feels, and it's also what they like to spread. They want the other person in their relationship to feel shame so they're embarrassed, confused, unsure about their behavior, and more likely to hand the control back over to them so they are in charge, as shown by this quote featured at ***After Narcissistic Abuse*** (at *afternarcissisticabuse.wordpress.com/2014/04/07/the-narcissistic-rage-cycle*):

"There is a saying that when you're a hammer the world looks like a nail. When you're a narcissist, the world looks like it should approve, adore, agree and obey you. Anything less than that feels like an assault and because of that a narcissist feels justified in raging back at it.

What is at the core of narcissists is not what is often referred to as low self-esteem. I don't think that is accurate, but something that the people around them say to themselves to mollify their own rage at the narcissist, i.e. "Oh, they only act that way, because they lack self-esteem."

What is really at the core of narcissists is an instability in their ability to feel and sustain feeling bigger, larger, smarter and more successful than everyone else which they need to feel stable. And just as Hamlet's mother said, "the lady doth protest too much," "the narcissist doth brag, scorn, talk down, primp and belittle too much" in order to continually prove to the world and themselves that they are larger than life. This is not to increase their self-esteem as much as it is to continually spackle the holes in their core that lead to a feeling of instability – and that, if not spackled, will lead to brittleness followed by fragmentation.

Narcissistic rage occurs when that core instability is threatened and furthermore threatened to destabilize them even further. Not unlike a wounded animal being the most vicious (because they think the next wound would kill them), narcissistic rage occurs when narcissists believe the next insult/assault to their grandiose based stability would shatter them.

In essence the reason narcissists are so self-centered is that their grandiosity-based center needs to be constantly reinforced to remain stable."

The first step to overcoming this shame, for the victim and the perpetrator, is **recognizing it for what it is**. When you see it coming, you can work out what your triggers are, how you immediately react when they crop up, and what happens next. Just noticing what's going on can lead to making some incredible, positive changes. This is something that we will go into more detail about in the following chapter.

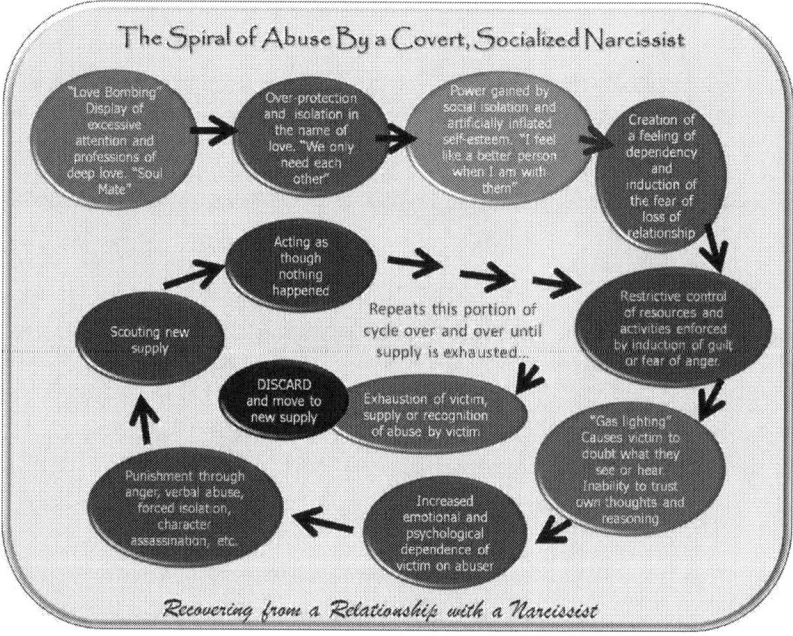

This is a cycle that starts off wonderfully with the 'love bombing' – an overwhelming amount of affection that borders on abnormal, but it quickly descends into isolation from everyone else in your life, a lot of self-doubt which includes the fear that you might be losing your mind completely, and ends in verbal and sometimes even physical abuse. This will only end if the victim walks away or the narcissist grows bored of the game.

3. Your Emotions

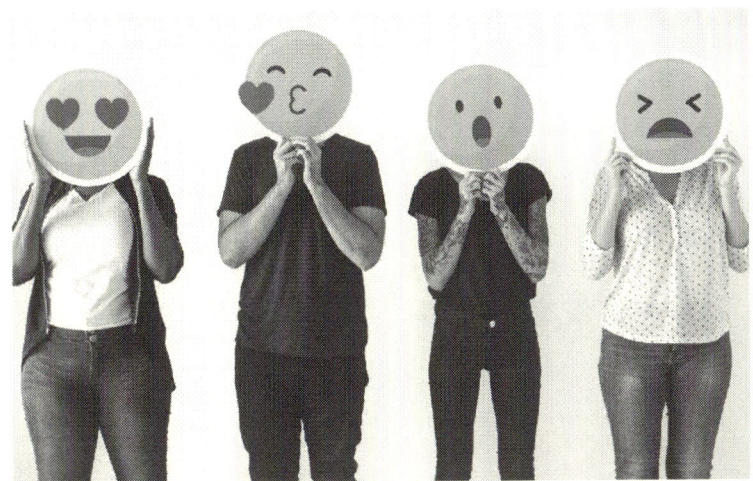

Being lied to a lot and pushed to one side while a narcissist takes full control all the time can damage you emotionally. That isn't always just an accidental thing. Even if the other person suffers from Narcissistic Personality Disorder, there are mind control tactics that they use purposefully to ensure that they are always the one in charge.

Here are **some examples as to what narcissists will do to disarm the other person**:

- The *assumption* – the narcissist will assume things, then speak about them as if they are the truth. This often leaves the victim confused and unable to argue.
- *Love bomb* – the victim will receive all kinds of compliments and loving feelings. These are to ensure that there are good times to look back on when times are bad.
- *Degradation* – backhanded compliments, small insults, little ways to damage the victim's self-confidence.
- *Emotional blackmail* – this might come in the form of verbal assaults, guilt, humiliation – anything to get what they want.
- *Shows of power* – demands, unpredictability, yelling – anything to show the other person that they are the one in charge.

It's like living in constant chaos, which is very unhealthy for everyone. Staying in that situation will just chip away at the victim until they are too emotionally drained to even consider fighting back anymore. The victim will become a shell of who they used to be, which needs to change.

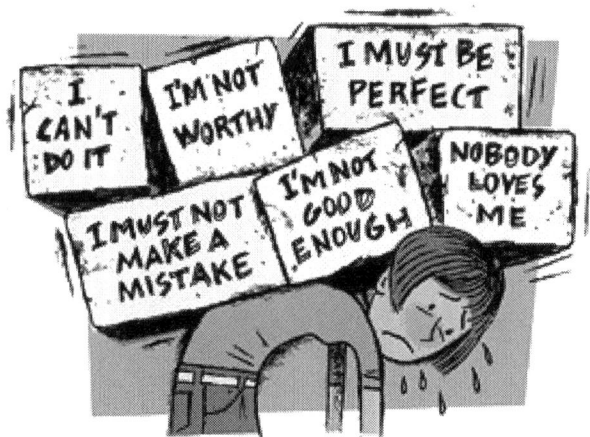

These are **the top fourteen signs identifying that your self-esteem is dangerously low**. Take a look to see if this applies to you:

- Anxiety and social withdrawal
- Emotional problems
- Low self-confidence, periods of sadness and depression
- Lack of social conformity
- Problems eating, even eating disorders
- Struggle accepting compliments from others
- Viewing yourself as worse than you actually are
- Hyper focus on negative aspects
- Exaggerating what you imagine other people are thinking
- Poor self-care habits, but taking care of others
- Always wondering if you have treated people badly
- Hesitate to accept challenges
- Lose the ability to trust in your own thoughts and opinions
- Stop expecting more from life

This list sounds exhausting to even read, never mind live through. If this is your life, then you really need to make some positive changes for yourself. You need to put yourself first for a change.

4. Your Conversations

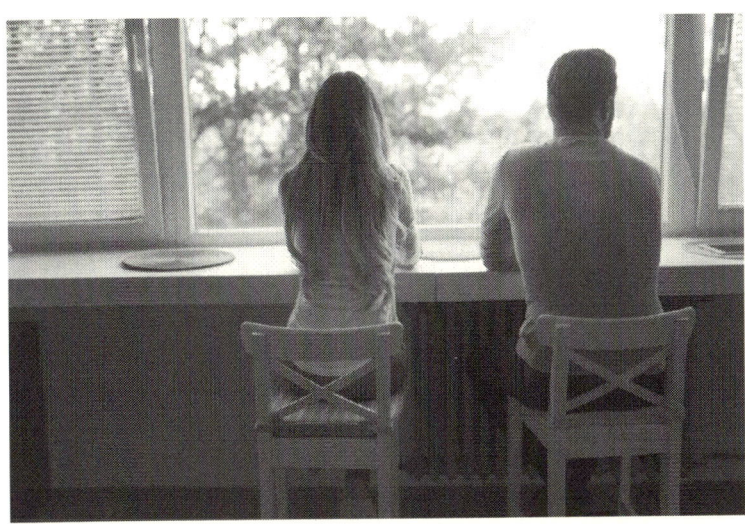

Talking to a narcissist isn't like talking to anyone else. Their toxic shame and weak ego mean they don't interact with people in a way that doesn't benefit them. That's because more often than not, they are dissociated in their mind. *Mind* (at www.mind.org.uk) explains this disorder further:

"Dissociation is one way the mind copes with too much stress, such as during a traumatic event. The word dissociation can be used in different ways but it usually describes an experience where you feel disconnected in some way from the world around you or from yourself.

If you dissociate for a long time, especially when you are young, you may develop a dissociative disorder. Instead of dissociation being something you experience for a short time it becomes a far more common experience and often the main way you deal with stressful experiences."

Some dissociative experiences include:	A doctor or psychiatrist might call these experiences:
• Having gaps in your life where you can't remember anything that happened • Not being able to remember information about yourself or about things that happened in your life	*Dissociative amnesia*

• Travelling to a different location and taking on a new identity for a short time (without remembering your identity)	*Dissociative fugue*
• Feeling as though the world around you is unreal • Seeing objects changing in shape, size and color • Seeing the world as 'lifeless' or 'foggy' • Feeling as if other people are robots (even though you know they're not)	*Derealization*
• Feeling as though you are watching yourself in a film or looking at yourself from the outside • Feeling as you are just observing your emotions • Feeling disconnected from parts of your body or your emotions • Feeling as if you are floating away • Feeling unsecure of the boundaries between yourself and other people	*Depersonalization*
• Your identity shifting and changing • Speaking in a different voice or voices • Using different name or names • Switching between different parts of your personality • Feel as if you are losing control to 'someone else'	*Identity alteration*

• Experience different parts of your identity at different times • Acting like different people, including children	
• Find it difficult to define what kind of person you are • Feeling as though there are different people inside you	*Identity confusion*

Here are some tips for **when you want to talk to a narcissist in a way that they will respond to positively**:

- Do not make demands of them and have no expectations.
- Prepare to listen to what they say.
- Look for ways to give them positive acknowledgement frequently.
- Be sincere and honest when you praise them.
- Try not to think about their ego. Talk to them in a way you know they'll respond to and understand.
- Avoid challenging what they want so they do not get defensive.
- If none of this works out, smile a lot and keep quiet.

This might sound like a lot of give and not much take, and that's because it is. But this is just a way to practice patience while you start on your breakthrough with them. This is a way to get them to do what you would like for once, such as getting some help.

Here are even more **tactics to help you get your own way for a change**:

- Use concise and clear language when you explain what you want.
- Be aware of what they want; be sure to acknowledge that during the conversation.
- Assure the narcissist that what you want will provide them a positive benefit, otherwise you'll never get their approval.

You need to start taking control of the conversation more so that you aren't railroaded into behaving in a certain way anymore. It isn't always easy, but the next chapter will give you some tools to help you with that.

5. Your Boundaries

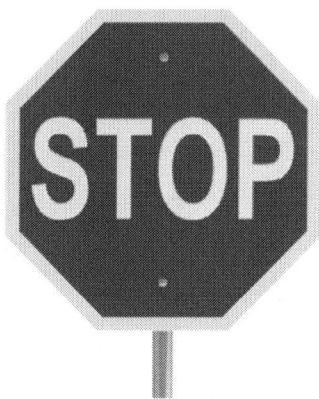

Everyone has their own set of personal boundaries; it's how we ensure that the people around us treat us with the respect that we deserve. Living with someone who constantly belittles us can shred these boundaries and leave us unsure of how we should be treated anymore. Losing our boundaries can be one of the worst side effects of narcissistic abuse, because it means the victim allows him or herself to be treated in ways that wouldn't normally happen. This is why the cycle continues for far too long.

Here are **some clues to look out for if you fear your boundaries aren't as healthy as they should be**:

- Your relationship is very dramatic and full of explosive situations.
- Decision-making is really hard, because you are unsure of what you need or want.
- You're a people pleaser, even when it means letting yourself down.
- You live in a cycle of guilt and anxiety.
- You're always tired for seemingly no reason. This is because you expend so much emotional energy.
- You don't know when to stop sharing – information, your things, everything is up for grabs.
- You are always a victim, feeling defeated, as if the world has it in for you.
- You are always edgy and annoyed. This is because you're constantly working against your own values.
- You want more respect, but you don't know how to get it.
- Passive aggression forms a lot of your communication.

- You don't know who you really are, which leaves you feeling lost.
- Your fear of rejection is overwhelming.

This can lead to **enmeshment**, which is defined by *Fuls Heart Transition* (at *fulsheartransition.com/enmeshment-symptoms-and-causes*) as:

"Enmeshment is a description of a relationship between two or more people in which personal boundaries are permeable and unclear. This often happens on an emotional level in which two people "feel" each other's emotions, or when one person becomes emotionally escalated and the other family member does as well. A good example of this is when a teenage daughter gets anxious and depressed and her mom, in turn, gets anxious and depressed. When they are enmeshed the mom is not able to separate her emotional experience from that of her daughter even though they both may state that they have clear personal boundaries with each other. Enmeshment between a parent and child will often result in over involvement in each other's lives so that it makes it hard for the child to become developmentally independent and responsible for her choices."

As you can see from this statement, it can be a good thing when both parties are happy, but when the narcissist isn't, there's a sense of love starvation, shame, fear, and no tolerance.

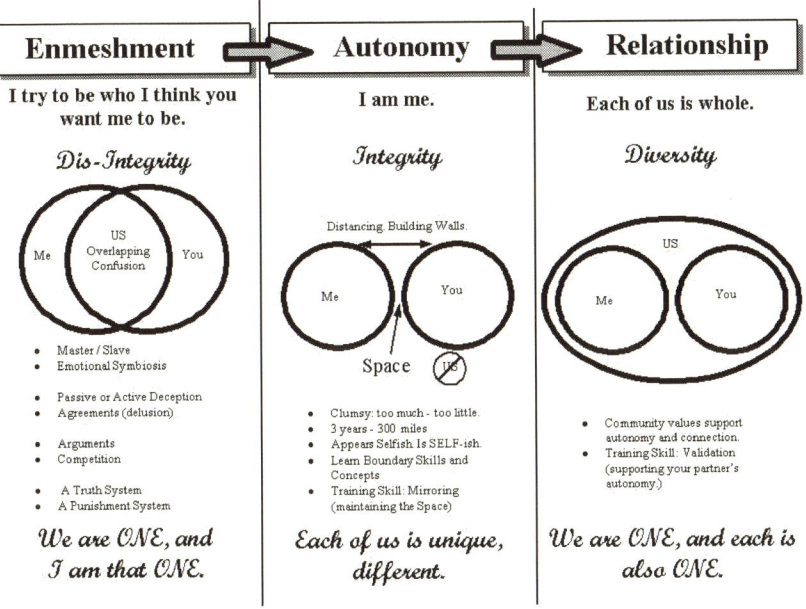

6. Your Image

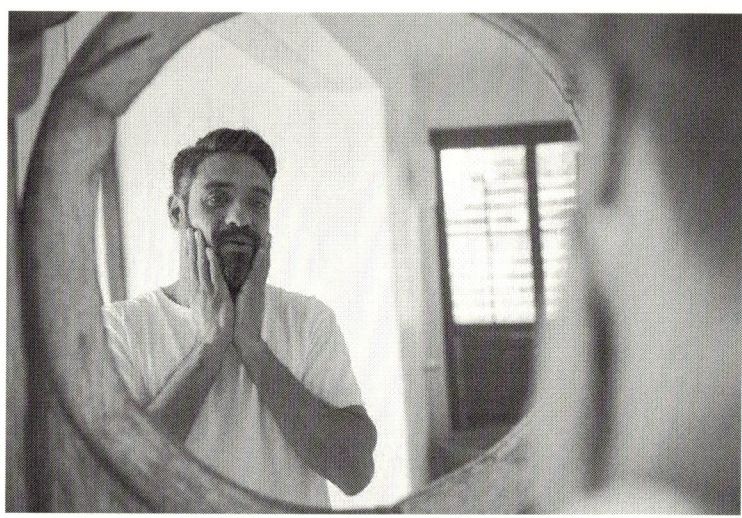

It's hard to imagine that being with someone narcissistic can actually affect the way you look, but it does. When you don't see yourself in the same way that you used to, you won't dress or make the same sort of effort with yourself. Maybe your narcissistic person doesn't want you to look your best, so for an easier life you make less effort, or maybe you are something to show off to the world so you always have to look your best.

It might not seem like much, it's just a change in the way that you dress, but this is something about you that's being controlled. The way that you look is a big part of you, and having that taken away is stripping you of a part of who you are, and it is something to worry about. Especially if you feel like you can't change that in the way that you want. There's something very wrong with the situation if you don't feel you can wear nice clothes and makeup, or even if you feel like you can't dress down. What you put on your body should be up to you, always!

STOP MANIPULATING ME!

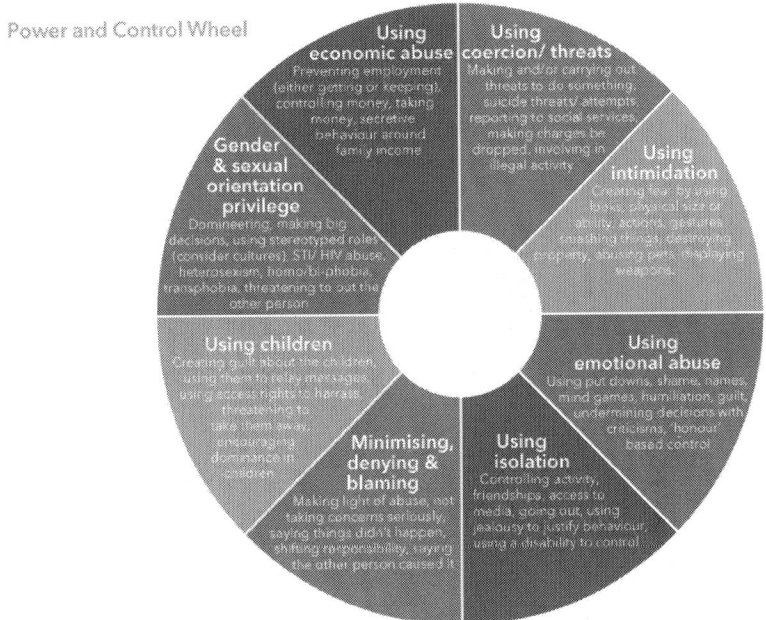

If you feel like your love is restricting you, then you need to get some help. If there isn't anyone in your family or friendship circle that you feel like you can trust, then there are a number of local services you can turn to for help. Emotional abuse is a form of abuse, whether it always seems like it or not.

7. Your Mind

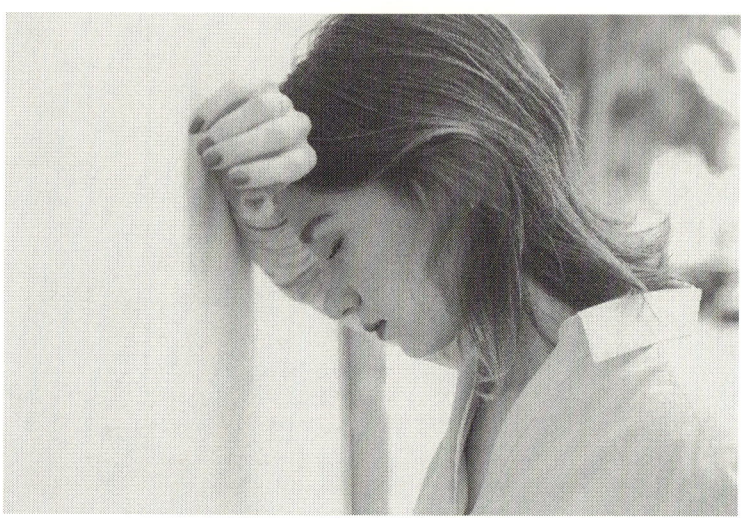

The effect that living with a narcissist can have on your psyche is deep-rooted and hard to extract yourself from. Recognizing it for what it is must be the first step towards getting away from it. Whether that means escaping it or helping the person out, first you need to identify the behavioral patterns. Whether it seems like it or not, it's mind control tactics.

This **mind control can come in a number of forms**:

- *Charm* – we've already looked at how charming these narcissists can be, creating good times so it isn't all bad. These events are probably constantly brought up whenever things aren't the greatest.
- *Personality Hijack* – if the person you live with is prone to explosive outbursts that come from situations that don't seem to call for it, you'll always be afraid and on edge.
- *Gaslighting* – this isn't an official psychology term, but one that's often used to describe narcissistic behavior. They lie all the time, and when they're discovered, they turn things around and make it seem like the victim is going crazy. They do this so well because they're wonderful at manipulation, especially with someone they know well.
- *Smear Campaign* – public humiliation is a terrible threat, and even worse when it's really happening. No one wants to be made to look foolish, which the narcissist uses against you. By making you look like the crazy, bad person, it makes it more challenging for you to say the truth without complying to this notion.

- *Triangulation* – by comparing you to other people, jealousy automatically rears its ugly head. It's hard to remain rational when you have envy inside of you.
- *Sabotage* – they might sabotage your career, your friendships, your family bonds, your self-esteem.
- *Withholding* – they might withhold love, sex, money, or anything that will make you feel neglected and isolated.
- *Nastiness* – comments, aggression, or even violence to ensure that you behave in a certain way will also be used.

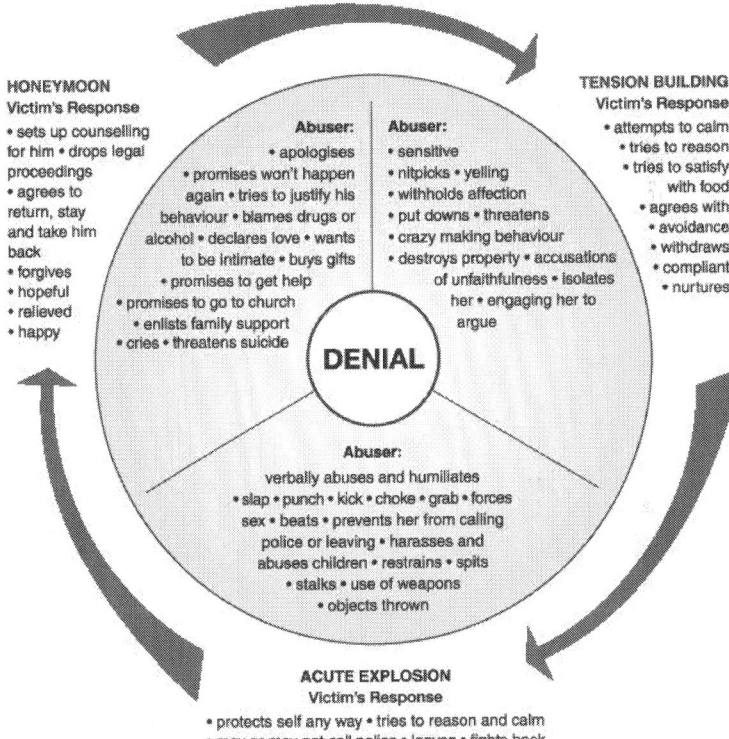

To help yourself get out of a situation where your mind has been controlled for a very long time, you need to ensure that you have some distance. It might be hard, but you have to extract yourself while you heal. Depending on how long you've been affected by this emotional abuse, you might even need to get some professional help from a licensed medical professional.

8. Your Environment

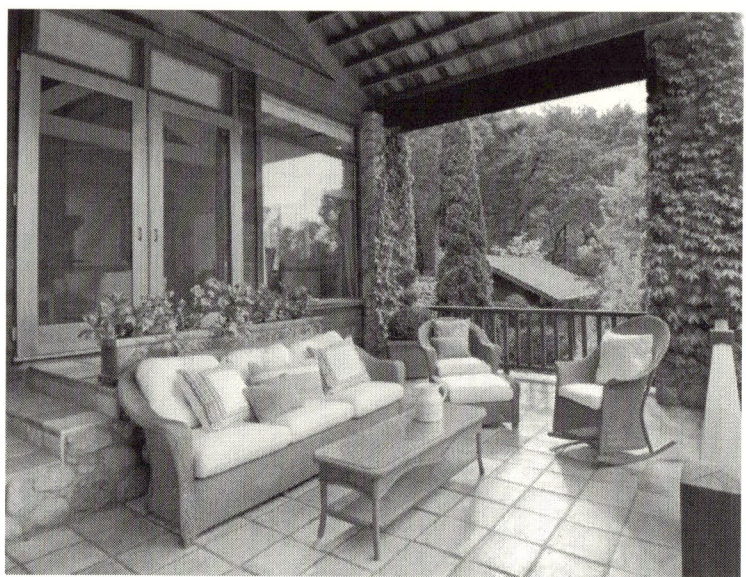

A narcissist has certain situations in which they thrive. They will be much more aggressive with their control in the home, where other people cannot see them being their worst. They will be much more likely to publicly humiliate you with people they feel comfortable with, because they know it'll be taken well by the audience. They even do well in the workplace, because their inflated sense of self-confidence ensures that other people see them as better than they are.

Here are **some examples of where certain types of narcissists feel at their most comfortable**:

- The *'know it all'* – this might be a friend or someone in the workplace. Either way, they constantly give you a whole load of 'helpful' advice even when it isn't needed. They can be fairly harmless, but very annoying, especially, when they act like they know everything and you don't.

- The *'grandiose'* – this is someone who acts more important than everyone. This person is usually in charge in the workplace, where they can lord their assumptions and self-importance over everyone else.

- The *'seductive'* – this is the sort of person you might find yourself in a relationship with. They will charm you with compliments and flattery, making you feel amazing about yourself. Of course, this doesn't last long. Soon, the cold shoulder will come out, leaving you desperate for that affection again.

- The *'bully'* – this person belittles everyone around them with horrible tactics. Name-calling, violence, aggression. Narcissist parents often behave this way.
- The *'vindictive'* – you cannot challenge this narcissist on their authority or they will set out to make your life a living hell. This could be someone that you work alongside, or a sibling or friend, who you are constantly competing with.

9. Your Body

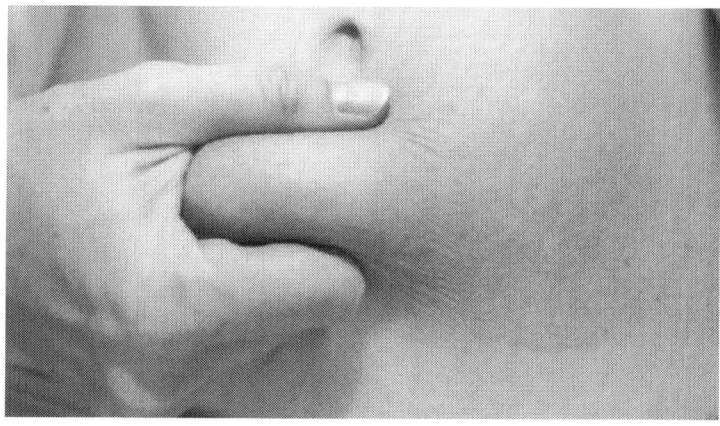

Your self-esteem has a dramatic effect on your body. If you have bad feelings about yourself psychologically, then your body begins to respond physically. As previously discussed, you won't dress in a way that makes you feel good about yourself, but it's more than that. The stress of living with someone who suffers from narcissism can change many different parts of you.

Here are **some of the most common examples of things you might notice**:

- Fatigue or low energy.
- Migraines and headache.
- Diarrhea, upset stomach, or sickness.
- Body and muscle pains and aches.
- Chest pain and a racing heartbeat.
- Insomnia or struggle getting to sleep.
- Heightened sensitivity to infections and the common cold.
- Lack of sexual desire.
- Chills, shakiness, and nervousness.
- Difficulty swallowing and dry mouth.
- Grinding teeth.
- Weight changes, this can be gain or loss.

These changes in your body are warning signs that something isn't right and that you need to get some help. Even starting with these ailments is a big step in the right direction.

10. Your Behavior

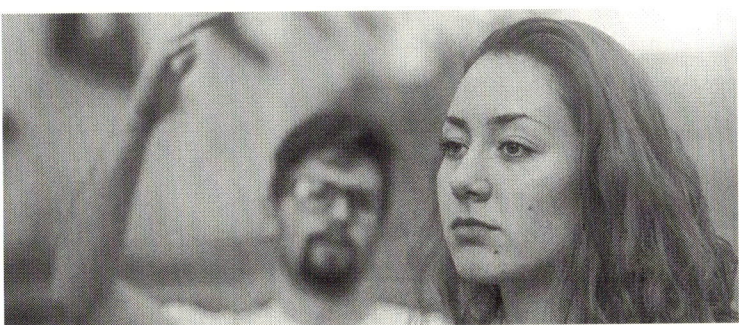

This isn't to say that your behavior is the reason for the emotional abuse, more that it changes because of it. When your self-esteem is being attacked on a daily basis, it's hard to remember how you once acted. You can become so stuck in the protective shell that you've put around yourself that you feel lost and you don't know who you are.

Maybe this is something that you need to discuss with other people. If you haven't isolated yourself from all your friends and family, you can ask them if they've noticed a difference in you. This can open an honest line of communication as to what they think the cause is and can be the first step in asking for some help to change.

If you wish to change the narcissist in your life, you first need to look at yourself. You are not responsible for how they behave, but you need to gather some inner strength before you can push for the positive changes that you need. There will be more detail in the actionable steps you can take for this in the next chapter of the book.

8 TIME-TESTED TACTICS TO OVERCOME NARCISSISM

1. Understand

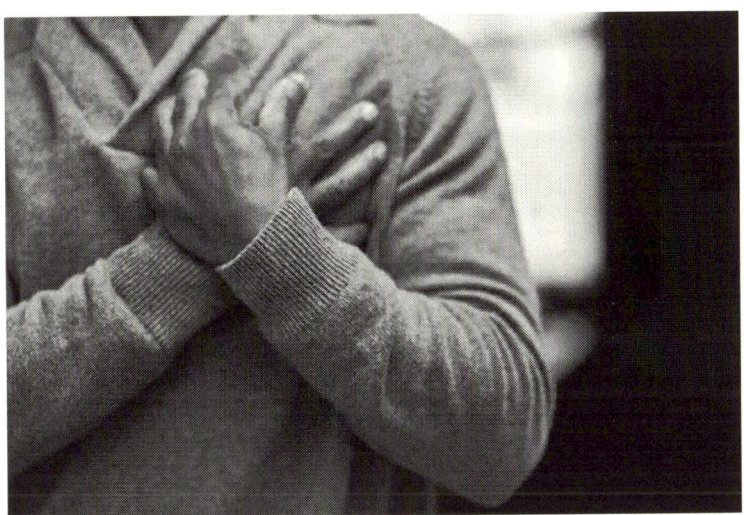

I know this might be hard to get your head around, but the first step to recover, no matter where on the narcissism scale the perpetrator is, is understanding. You need to find out *where* the narcissism has come from and why it makes the person act in the way that they do. As we've seen throughout this book, a lot of this behavior is learned from a negative childhood. While this might not make it any better now, having an understanding will help you with the following steps.

If, after reading the last chapter, you have identified that you are living with a narcissist, and you want to understand them, you'll need to have an open and honest conversation with them about their life and behavior. This won't be easy and will take a lot of patience on your behalf, but if you're serious about breaking the negative cycle of your life, then it's something you need to do.

Here are **some tips to help you with this**:

- Don't worry about arguing who is right and wrong. This isn't the time or place for it, and you probably won't win. Bringing up their defenses helps no one.
- Empathize with how they are feeling. Narcissists love being understood, even if they don't offer the same courtesy back.
- Instead of saying *'I feel disappointed...'* try *'I know you feel disappointed when...'*
- Take responsibility. If you show you're willing to accept your part of the blame, they might be more keen to do the same.
- When digging into the past, don't ask directly; use a more roundabout method by either asking for advice or going in with a topic that they enjoy speaking about.
- Compliment them as you talk. Especially if they start discussing difficulties from their past. Make sure they know that you admire them for what they've been through.

Once you learn more about where this negative behavior has come from, you can start identifying it when it crops up again. Here are **some ideas of the sorts of things you might want to look out for**:

- Rejection.
- Someone leaving.
- Helplessness over painful situations.
- Being ignored or someone being unavailable.
- Disapproval, blame, or shame.
- Someone blaming or shaming you.
- Losing control.

So, while talking to the narcissist about their behavioral patterns is the best place to start on this journey, it might not be the most effective way to understand. A conversation, however well-intentioned and well thought out it might be, can bring out the defensive side in a narcissist. You can also use what you already know about the person, and you can talk to the other people in their lives to find out more about them. This can be close friends or other family members, maybe even people from their past. Anyone who knows the narcissist and might be able to shed some productive insight into why they are acting the way that they are.

However you can discover the source of the person's narcissism, do it.

This journey into understanding the narcissist isn't to make you feel sympathy for them, it's to help you understand yourself better and why you keep getting trapped by them. It'll also make it so much clearer that you aren't to blame for everything that's happened, and that their behavior is actually only about them.

Another positive outcome of this is that by talking to others you will see that you aren't alone, that there are others who have been through the same at their hand. Gaining some allies and having some people on your side will assist you in building up the strength that you really need to move on.

2. Acknowledge

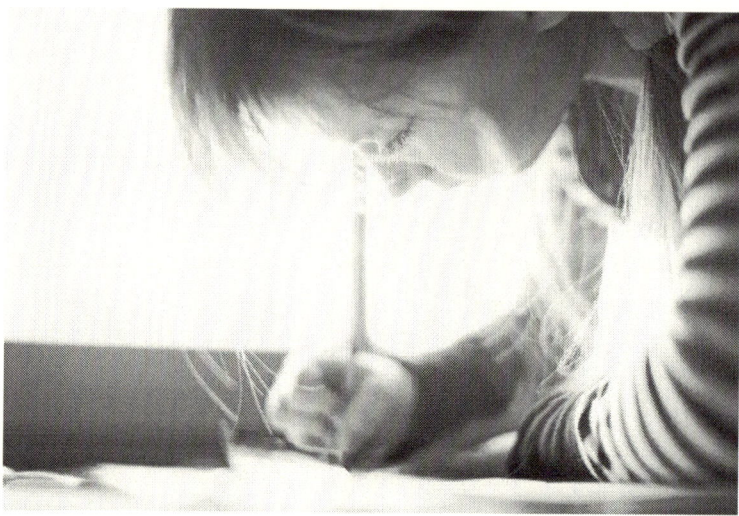

Now it is time to acknowledge, which means there's no more burying your head in the sand. You need to fully accept everything that's happened and any role that you might have played in that. That doesn't mean continue to blame yourself for things that aren't your fault, but accept when you haven't always reacted in the best way possible. This also means acknowledging that you have spotted these negative patterns in the past but that you've ignored them, because that's an important step in moving forward now.

Here are **some great tips to help you with this stage**:

- Use cool processing – think about *why* events made you feel a certain way, rather than *what* they made you feel. This will help you to understand the way that you've been living for however long the narcissistic cycle has been happening.
- Personalize, don't generalize – every situation is different, every person who suffers from narcissism is unique, and so is the victim. Remember that as you acknowledge what has happened.
- Practice self-compassion – don't judge yourself as you move forward because that only holds the process up. Accepting yourself wholly, including the mistakes you've made and the bad behavior that you've accepted for far too long, will only help you to move on.
- Take the high road – if things get messy when you're finally regaining some of your courage, remember not to get sucked in by pettiness. You're moving on now, not getting stuck in the past.

You might find it helpful to write everything down while you're going through this, and that includes everything that you've learned while you've been understanding the narcissist, just because having things on paper can make them feel much more real.

Write down why the person is a narcissist, what brought you into their life in the first place, and why you're still around now. What keeps you there? Why haven't you left yet? While you're figuring that out, it can also be helpful to figure out what triggers the narcissist and how that makes you feel inside. Figuring out this negative pattern will assist you in breaking free from it. Make a note of everything that you think is important, maybe even write it as a letter to the narcissist – even if you don't send it. It can be a cathartic exercise.

Here are some tips for you on **how to accept things successfully**:

- Not punishing yourself for how bad things have become.
- Letting go of the negative cycle and how it makes you feel.
- Disengaging from the narcissistic patterns.
- Not expecting anything from the other person.
- Not getting bogged down in agreeing or disagreeing with what's happened.
- Acknowledging and accepting in a calm way.
- Allowing the things you cannot control to just be as they are.

Here is **some helpful advice for starting to get your life back as you want it**:

- Set a realistic goal – things won't ever be exactly as they were before because you and the world have both changed.
- Get rid of toxicity – move past anything or anyone negative because this only brings you down and distorts how you see yourself.
- Stop believing that you can't do it. You *do* have the strength.

Once you feel like you've fully acknowledged what has happened while you've been trapped in this vicious cycle, and this is something that you've accepted and come to terms with at least somewhat, then it's time to move on to the next step, which is all about restoring wholeness in your life. You have more than likely existed without this narcissistic person in your life and you were someone. You need to work on getting back to that person, or as close as you can be. It might be a slow process, but it's a worthwhile one.

3. Disarm

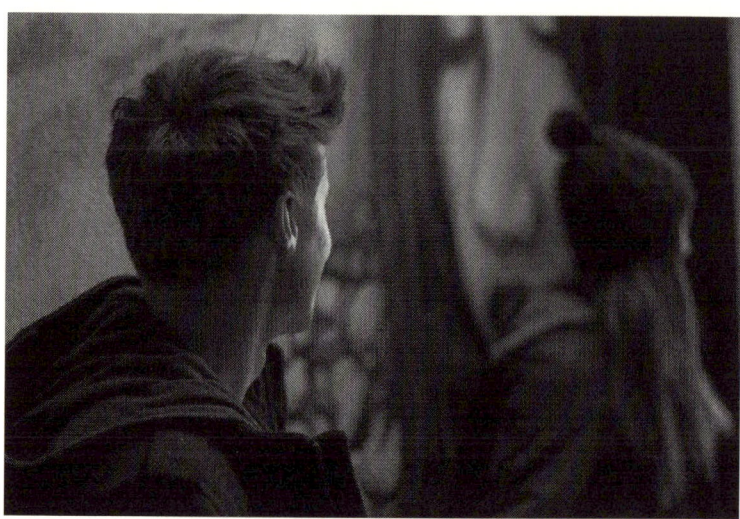

You have spent a lot of your time being disarmed by a narcissist, which is why you're trapped in their bubble. They have used mind control and manipulation techniques, discussed in one of the early chapters of this book, to make you feel like you have been in the wrong the entire time, probably leading you to question your own sanity along the way. Well, now it's time for you to do the disarming. You'll need to still use some flattery and be careful with your wording, but it's very possible to do, and it's also a great start to regaining the control. Not necessarily control over them but over yourself and the way that you behave.

To start feeling differently and acting in a new way, you need to change the way that you deal with that person. But you have to do it in the right way so it doesn't spiral and cause arguments and defensive behavior that doesn't help anyone. You don't want to get caught up in the cycle any longer; you're now trying to pull away from it.

Here are **some great tips to help you with this**:

- Disengage – don't pay attention to the bait that's being thrown your way. Rise above it and ignore it because you don't want to get sucked back in.

"I refuse to discuss this right now..."

- Build up your walls – know what you want and don't let anyone overstep that. This might be scary to start with, but will end up with you gaining more respect for yourself.

"I would appreciate it if you didn't do that again..."

- Stop apologizing – you are not always the one in the wrong! Let them know that they cannot control your emotions anymore; they can't force you to feel guilt any longer.

"I do not believe I am the one to blame..."

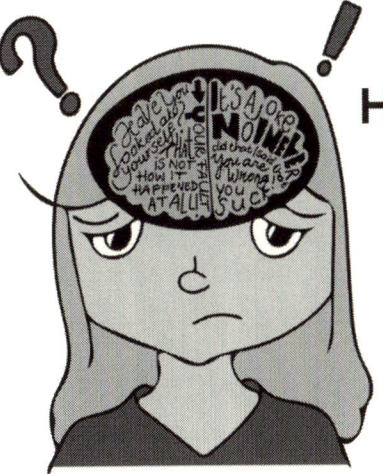

How to Deal with Gaslighting & Crazy-Making

More on what it is, how it works, and what to do about it on: swanwaters.com/gaslighting

What To Do:

> Realize that you are not responsible for someone else's behavior.

> Talk about the episode to those you trust.

> Journaling can help to keep track of what actually happened and help you not to get lost is the abuser's version of reality. Make sure the journal is kept private.

> Remember you will never win a debate with this person as they are so convincing and persistently right, they'll run rings around you.

> Keep a record, especially in the workplace where the abuse may lead to legal action.

> If any events escalate to violence find safety, and then report it to the police immediately.

What Not To Do:

> Don't take responsibility or blame for what they are feeling.

> Don't make snap judgments of others just because you have heard bad things about them.

> Don't engage in arguments with a Toxic Person or abuser, or try to convince them you are right.

> If you feel unsafe either physically, emotionally or verbally then get help to leave!

> Don't keep secrets, find someone to share your experience with.

In fact, there is one study that shows **the five key phrases identified to always disarm a narcissist**. Try them out and see if they work:

- *I am sorry you feel that way.*
- *I can accept your faulty perception of me.*
- *I have no right to control how you see me.*
- *I guess I have to accept how you feel.*
- *Your anger is not my responsibility.*

This is all about empowering yourself and reminding yourself that you are worthwhile. You've probably spent far too much time being put down and made to feel insignificant by the narcissist, because that's the emotional state that they need you to be in so they can keep controlling you. Those feelings of guilt and shame aren't really yours, so you can let go of them if you allow yourself to.

While you disarm your narcissist you also need to take care of yourself so you are healthy and able to move forward successfully when the time feels right. There is no rush to make this happen; you have to do it on your own timescale, or you'll only end up back in the same position that you were in before. This can involve taking some space for yourself, doing little things that benefit only you (which you probably haven't done in a very long time), or even just talking with a friend. Anything that will help you feel better and stronger in yourself will assist you in the long run.

No one can empower you but – YOU – and once you have empowered yourself...

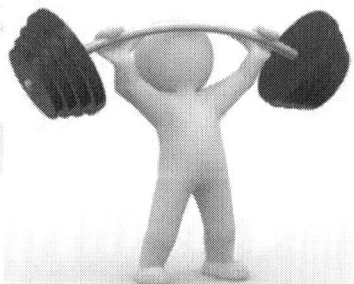

No one can take that power away.

4. React Differently

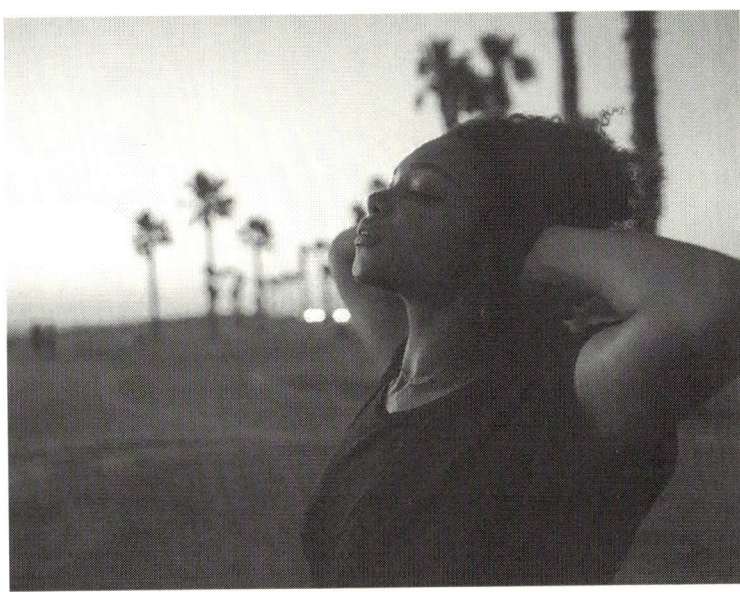

It's important to remember that it isn't your fault; there is nothing you can do about someone who has narcissistic tendencies. I hope that's something you've learned while understanding and acknowledging the situation. They can only change if they want to, but you are in control of your own behavior. It probably hasn't felt that way for a while, but you are. You need to get back behind the driver's seat of how you behave to make some positive changes.

Here are **some tips for helping you to take back control of yourself and your life**:

- **Be selfish** – start thinking about what *you* want. You've lived your life for someone else for such a long time; it's time to reclaim your identity. As stated in the previous part of this chapter, do some things that are just for you.
- **Say 'no'** – the narcissist might not be used to hearing it, but you need to stop giving in to the other person's demands. It won't be easy, but you have to do this if you want your life back. If you do not wish to do something, then don't – even if you know it'll make your life harder. This will only be temporary because eventually the cycle will be broken completely.
- **Step away** – you'll need to take a step away from the situation to move on. Whether you want to stay with the narcissist or not, you need to step back while you both change your behaviors. This will in-

volve taking some real space from one another, and if they don't want to accept this, *you* have to be the one to enforce it.

- **Stop making excuses** – don't think of reasons to stay and to keep living in the vicious cycle. There are reasons why a narcissist behaves like they do, but that's not an excuse to stay as they are. There are ways the person can change; they just need to do it. *You* cannot control that.
- **Look forward** – stop focusing on the past, or you won't be able to move on with your life. Don't start dwelling on only the good times, because they are always littered with the bad and going back can easily result in you sliding back into that cycle.

Saying 'no' is probably the hardest thing on this list, at least to start with, so here are **some helpful ways to start practicing saying no in a nice way**:

- *Not right now.*
- *I don't want to do that.*
- *That isn't going to work out for me.*
- *Let me get back to you about that.*
- *Can I get back to you?*
- *Oh, I wish I could!*
- *Right now I have other things that I need to focus on.*

You don't have to say it in a direct and nasty-sounding way, but you do need to start saying it somehow. Practice it as much as you can. The more you say it, the easier it will become, and you'll soon realize how much you benefit from all the free time you now have not focusing on other people.

All of this is challenging the psychological cage that you've been trapped in for quite some time, so of course that isn't going to be straightforward. It's easier in the short term to keep things as they are, because breaking routine and disrupting the flow of things can cause a massive life upheaval, but it's this upheaval that you need. In the long term, it will be really beneficial to you. Having allies and other people that you can rely on will stop you feeling isolated and give you strength.

Often the reason people cannot face change is because they do not feel like they have anyone to help them. If this is the case for you, and you do not feel like you have anyone to turn to, look up available organizations in your area. There's no reason for you to face this completely by yourself.

5. Stop Playing

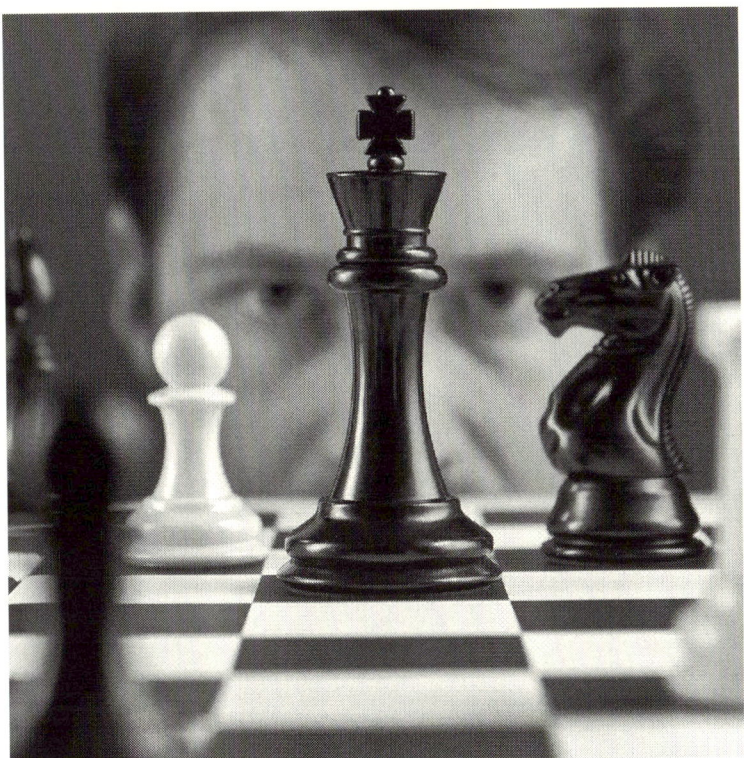

The vicious cycle that you've been existing in is a game. Not to you, but to the narcissist. They've been manipulating you and all the situations that you've been through like a puppet controlling your strings, and enjoying the journey along the way. Even the challenges you've put up to them have probably been a part of the fun for them as they try to bring you back down once again. You *need* to stop playing. The only way to protect yourself is to extract yourself from the game completely.

Here are **some great examples of the games you've been involved in**:

- **Ping Pong** – the back and forth between you and the narcissist, where any accusation you fling at them is sent back with a million and one excuses, is exhausting. That's why you *have* to stop getting sucked into arguments.
- **Gotcha!** – you've been fed a lot of phony affection, empathy, and love. When this gets pulled away suddenly, you don't know where you stand anymore. You need to recognize what emotions are genuine and fake so you can't get tricked again.

- ***Crazy Eights*** – a narcissist likes to call you crazy so you doubt your own sanity. They do it in such a way that it leaves you dizzy – *but* you do know your own mind. You are certain of what you know. Take a step back and recognize that you are smart and not crazy!
- ***Death by a Thousand Cuts*** – narcissists love to destroy your soul, your ego, your accomplishments. This is the sort of thing you have to ignore. It takes thick skin, but after everything you've endured, you can do this.
- ***Twenty-One*** – you're always treated like you're a child, patronized no matter what. You need to stand up for yourself and remember that you have your own mind.
- ***King and Queens Game*** – someone is always in charge; there's always a winner. Even if you don't know the rules, you can be penalized for breaking them. Refusing to acknowledge that the game even exists is the first step towards getting away from it.
- ***Cat and Mouse*** – the narcissist is always nipping at the tail of the victim, leaving them with no privacy. The only way to stop that would be to set up and maintain your personal boundaries.
- ***Poker*** – the lying with a straight face is something the narcissist is excellent at. If you really think about it, you do know what's the truth and what isn't. You just need to start owning that knowledge.

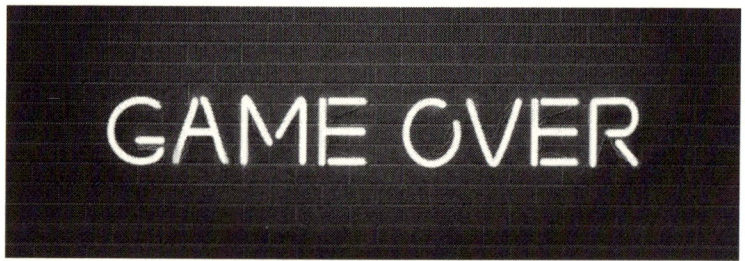

There are many ways in which you can **disengage from the narcissist**; we have already discussed 'saying no' to them and reacting differently in a previous part of this chapter, but now you need to think about *really* taking yourself away. By disengaging, you have to stop caring what they think about you, their words must affect you much less, and you cannot be afraid of them anymore. By not worrying about them, you inadvertently completely take the control back, which of course is exactly what you want.

Here are **some useful tips to help you with this**:

- Ground yourself in reality. Stop doubting yourself; you *know* what the truth is. A narcissist is wonderful at convincing you that their 'reality' is correct, so if this is something you struggle with, then give yourself evidence. Write things down as they happen or take photographs.

- Don't let them project their guilt or shame onto you. If you know something isn't your fault, simply refuse to accept it however much it winds them up. A strong support network is useful for this.

- The same goes for their exaggerations. By now, you know that they retell stories to make themselves look better and everyone else look worse. Simply reject things that they tell you if this crops up.

- Ignore them if they move the goalposts. Narcissistic people need to starve you of love so you're always chasing after it. Even if you do everything that they want all the time, it isn't good enough for them. Knowing that it never will be takes you one step closer to letting go of this and giving up the game completely. It's a pointless one anyway, and you'll never win it.

- If they change the subject all the time, especially when you're trying to communicate something important, don't give up. Keep on saying what you need to say. Maybe they'll never *really* hear it, but there are times when you just need to try.

- Maybe they will resort to name-calling and insults to get your attention, but this is only to cause you to react. The less visible reaction you make (even if it hurts inside), the quicker the narcissist will see that they're losing control of you.

- Smear campaigns may follow, where the narcissist doesn't tell you what they think of you, but they try to muddy your name instead. This is hard because the temptation can be to fight back, but this is what they want. Instead, hold your head high, ignore it all, and know that the important people in your life know the truth. However hard it is, this challenging time cannot last forever.

Once you stop playing these games, you will undoubtedly feel a sense of relief. You've spent too much of your time and effort trying to please someone who doesn't want to be pleased by you, they simply want to control you. No longer giving in to that is a really freeing sensation, but your work isn't over yet. Now you need to start really thinking about what to do next. The only way you can do that is by getting some distance, which is covered in the next part.

6. Separate

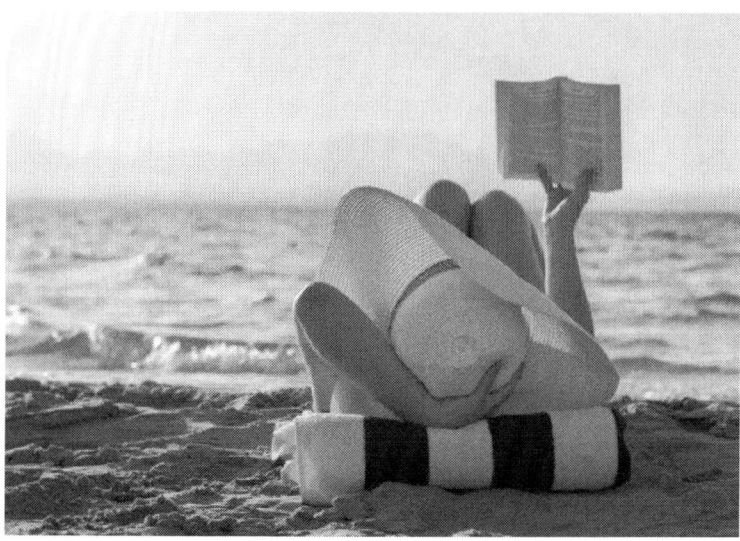

This doesn't necessarily mean you have to split up with the narcissist for good. It doesn't have to be *that* dramatic, but you will need some space to yourself while you both change your behavior. It's almost impossible to get out of a vicious cycle while you're still living together in the same environment, doing the same things. You need a fresh start.

Maybe this will lead to a full-time separation, if that's what's best for you or maybe even both of you, but that's something you won't find out for sure until you give it a try.

Getting this **temporary separation** while you're trying to work out your next steps can be difficult because it isn't always agreed with, which is why you need to make sure the distance is worthwhile. Here are **some tips to help you with this**:

- Have no contact the entire time. This is a proper break while you both work on yourselves. You don't want to be so focused on each other that nothing changes.
- Tell all your mutual friends that you don't want to know what's going on with the other person. The narcissist might act out in a disrespectful way and that information isn't helpful.
- Keep busy; don't give yourself time to grieve too much. Being alone with your thoughts can be very dangerous.

- Write everything in the form of a letter to your spouse. This isn't something you necessarily want to send, but you need to get it off your chest somehow.
- Don't fall for any manipulations; you *need* this time apart. Both of you do.
- Set limits and stick to them. You need a certain amount of time apart, so don't go back too soon.

This time won't be easy; it's going to be you unpacking a lot of learned behavior and habits that you've developed in order to create an easier life for yourself, but chances are that you've lost yourself along the way. But, it doesn't all have to be bad. You can also use this time to reconnect with people that you've let go along the way and restore those lost relationships. Family members, old friends, people that you've missed. You need to remind yourself who you really are. And you'll also need to **recover from these potential emotions**:

- Anxiety and panic
- Sleeplessness
- General fear and easily being scared
- External triggers that will remind you of the strained relationship you just had
- Struggling to maintain relationships
- Psychological and emotional numbness

You might even need to get some professional help with this, especially depending on how much time you've spent trapped in a narcissistic cycle. You may be so dragged down by the situation that you need to seek medical help, but even if you don't feel like you're at that stage, then it's good to have people who care about you around you – people who will ensure that you remain accountable and separate for the time that you're supposed to, even when you're feeling weak. Use this time to look inwards instead, disengage with them, and re-engage with yourself instead.

7. Heal

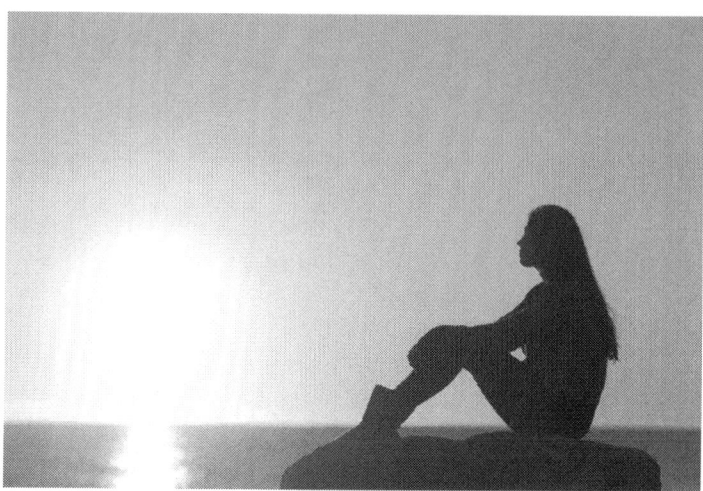

Once you've had your time apart, and you've worked out what you want to do next, it's time to start the healing process. Whether you chose to move back into your relationship with a brand-new attitude or move away into something different just for yourself, the healing process still needs to happen. You *have* to go through this step to get a much brighter future.

Here are **some great tips to help you with this**:

- Ground and soothe yourself. Try meditating and speaking to yourself much more kindly than you did before. You need to keep your self-confidence sky high.

- Allow yourself to feel all the emotions you need to feel. You might be angry, you might be sad, you might be elated for some space. You've been restricted for so long that now you can just feel.

- Seek help. Get some therapy either alone or together. Get an outside perspective on how to keep moving forward in a positive manner.

Through all of this, you *must* protect your boundaries. Whether together or alone, you need to take what you've learned during your time apart and keep it going. Remind yourself of the things that are important to you, even if you need to have Post-it notes or phone alerts to reiterate this. This might be personal space or private access to your online accounts; this could be a refusal to be spoken to negatively or even just time alone. Whatever's important to you, make it happen in a new relationship or in the same one. Don't fall back into the same patterns or all of this work becoming less susceptible to narcissism and the manipulation techniques used will have been for nothing.

CHOOSE YOUR RELATIONSHIPS WISELY. BEING ALONE WILL NEVER CAUSE AS MUCH LONELINESS AS BEING IN THE WRONG RELATIONSHIP.

via thisislovelifequotes.com

Sticking to the newer person that you've become can be just as hard as actually making the change, but with the right attitude you can move towards a brighter future. Here are **some tips to help keep you headed on the right path**, even when things feel at their toughest:

- Keep setting yourself positive, realistic goals to keep you moving forwards. Ensure you do all the things that you've always wanted to do but haven't been able to until now.
- Address any negativity in an instant so it doesn't become a toxic cycle again.
- Use motivational music or videos, or have a good friend or a counselor to talk to, to boost you up when things get tough. This will drag you from the black hole before it swallows you up.
- Learn to stay calm, find ways to control yourself and your own emotions.
- Change your perspective – you've done some really hard work on yourself; don't let that go.

8. Restore

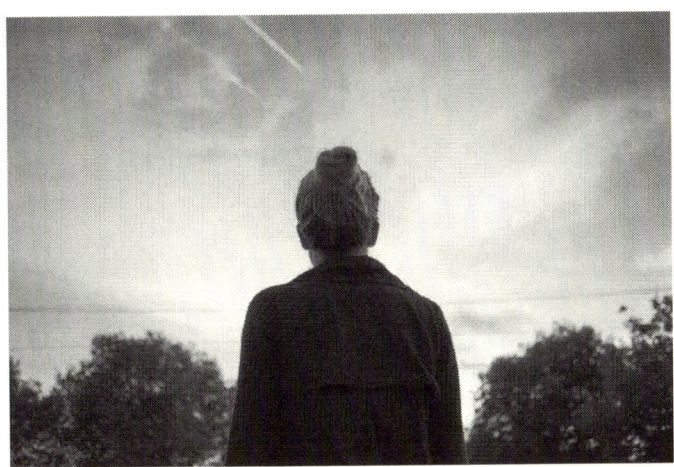

The final thing that you need to do is restore some sort of order in your life. You've had your space, you've worked out what you need to do, and now you've started to move forward with your life. Eventually, restoring order needs to happen in some form or another. You need to continue living your life. This will involve some building of a new identity, but that doesn't mean giving up being you. If anything, you'll be introducing more of yourself to the world.

Here are **some ideas to help you with this**:

- Use a calendar to schedule in the time for things you *need* to include in your new life. You don't want to forget or slide back into old, unhealthy patterns.

- Stick to this schedule no matter what. Don't let yourself slip back into old habits, especially, if you have returned to your relationship.

- Have someone to be accountable to. Someone who will let you know if things are going wrong again. Friends or family are perfect for this – as long as you listen to them.

- Take care of yourself. Don't allow yourself to slip back into any sort of negative cycles. Whether you are single or not, you are now the one in control. Don't let things slip backwards.

- Keep time for yourself set aside. Whether you go back to the relationship, you spend time being mostly alone, or you move on to new relationships, keep time for yourself because that's important in maintaining who you are. Allowing yourself to get swallowed up in someone else's personality and life is what landed you in the mess in the first place. *You* are special too; do not forget that, no matter what happens.

It might feel strange, living life as normal after such a massive upheaval, but hopefully, by this point, you've discovered new ways to live your life and be yourself. You've had a little bit of time being selfish and reminding yourself that you matter too, so keep that at the forefront as you live and grow. Whatever decision you make with regards to your relationship with the narcissist, there will be bumps in the road, but you have come this far and you *can* keep on going. Just make sure that you constantly remind yourself of that!

GLOSSARY

Here is **a glossary of terms to help you better understand yourself and the narcissist in your life**:

ACoNs

This acronym stands for "adult children of narcissists." It is commonly used by narcissism survivors and those who work with them.

Cluster B Personality Disorders

Personality disorders are grouped into three clusters by mental health professionals. Four Cluster B disorders are defined in the DSM-V (Diagnostic and Statistical Manual of Mental Disorders (fifth edition)), including histrionic personality disorder, borderline personality disorder, antisocial personality disorder, and narcissistic personality disorder. Often, an individual with one personality disorder will exhibit traits of one or more other disorders, a condition known as comorbidity.

Cognitive Dissonance

The narcissist's externalized, manufactured identity is built on lies and denial, and he/she expects his/her family members to accept his/her version of the "truth." What this means for the narcissist's spouse and children is that they find themselves in "opposite land," where he/she tells them (usually through a range of manipulative tactics) that "reality" is different from or even the opposite of what they feel and perceive. The narcissist produces a cognitive dissonance in others, who experience a profoundly disorienting gap between what they perceive and what the narcissist says happened – black is white, good is bad, false is true. Particularly in young children, cognitive dissonance is extremely traumatic, leading to self-doubt and disassociation.

C-PTSD

This stands for Complex Post-Traumatic Stress Disorder, a condition common in narcissistic abuse victims, as well as in people with NPD. C-

PTSD includes a wide range of disabling symptoms, including some or all of the following disturbances:
- hyper vigilance;
- generalized fear, anxiety, and agitation;
- over reactivity;
- insomnia;
- nightmares and/or night terrors;
- self-isolation;
- difficulty trusting;
- self-destructive behavior; and
- intrusive thoughts.

Denial

A person in denial willfully believes or pretends that traumatic events or circumstances do not exist or did not happen, oftentimes, even when presented with evidence to the contrary.

Devaluation

Because of their emotionally primitive perfect-or-worthless thinking (stuck at the developmental level of a young child) and their insistence on unattainable perfection, narcissists in relationships (with partners, family members, or friends) nearly inevitably become disillusioned. And because they lack a moral compass (again, like the stunted children they are), they do not hesitate to express their disappointment in a range of devaluing hostile behaviors, including judgment, belittlement, and rage, if not outright abandonment.

Divide and Conquer

This is a primary strategy narcissists use to assert control, particularly within their family, to create divisions among individuals. This weakens and isolates family members, making it easier for the narcissist to manipulate and dominate. The narcissist sets up an environment of competition and terror in which individuals are trying to avoid attack, often at one another's expense. He favors some and scapegoats others, breeding mistrust and resentment among siblings or between his spouse and children. Such dynamics also can play out in a work setting, where a boss uses the same kinds of tactics to control and manipulate his employees.

Enabler

Usually a partner/spouse of the narcissist, enablers "normalize" and even perpetuate the narcissist's grandiose persona, extreme sense of entitlement, and haughty attitude and behavior toward others by absorbing the abuse and acting as an apologist for it. Enablers are always avoiding conflict and attacking, while at the same time seeking rewards such as affection, praise, power, gifts, or money. Enablers may be under the delusion that they are the only ones who can truly understand the narcissist and oftentimes sacrifice or scapegoat their children to placate the narcissist.

Fauxpology

Because narcissists refuse accountability and believe they are always right, they rarely, if ever, genuinely apologize. Instead, they may toss out a false apology, or fauxpology, meant to deflect, induce guilt, or antagonize. Examples: "I'm sorry you think I'm such a disappointment as a mother," "I'm sorry you interpreted something so innocent as unfair," "I'm sorry you are so sensitive," "I'm sorry you can't understand how others feel," or "I'm sorry you are so angry."

Flying Monkeys

Just like the creatures serving the Wicked Witch in the film *The Wizard of Oz*, flying monkeys in the narcissistic family are enablers who help with the narcissist's dirty work, often to avoid being targeted themselves and/or to benefit from a certain level of bestowed privilege. The ones who are easily manipulated make the best flying monkeys. They may be children or other relatives.

Gaslighting

This is a form of psychological abuse in which narcissists systematically undermine other people's mental state by leading them to question their perceptions of reality. Narcissists use lies and false information to erode their victims' belief in their own judgment and, ultimately, their sanity. Common gaslighting techniques come in the form of denying and projecting: After an abusive incident, narcissists refuse responsibility, blame the abused, or outright deny that the abuse took place. They may say things like, "You're too sensitive," "You're crazy," "That's not what happened," "Why can't you let anything go," or "You made me do it." The term gaslighting comes from the 1944 Hollywood film *Gaslight*, a classic depiction of this kind of brainwashing.

Golden Child

This is a child singled out unfairly for favoritism, such as special privileges, more attention, high regard, exemption from discipline, and exemption from certain chores and responsibilities. Such favoritism is typically at the direct expense of a disfavored, scapegoated child.

Gray Rock

Going "gray rock" is a boundary-setting and conflict-avoidance strategy that can be effective in dealing with narcissists. It simply means making yourself dull and nonreactive, like a colorless unmoving rock. In gray-rock mode, you engage minimally with the narcissist and his/her circus of enablers/flying monkeys. You do not show or share your thoughts or feelings. You do not react to antagonism and manipulation. In short, you make yourself of little interest to the narcissist.

Hoovering

Since narcissists are by nature pathologically self-centered and often stunningly cruel, they ultimately make those around them unhappy, if not miserable, and eventually drive many people away. If people pull away or try to go no contact, narcissists may attempt to hoover (as in vacuum suck) them back within their realm of control. They try to hoover through a variety of means, from promising to reform their behavior, to acting unusually solicitous, to dangling carrots such as gifts or money. However, if they find replacement sources of supply, they may simply walk away from old ones.

Hypervigilance

To cope with a chaotic and often psychologically and physically abusive environment, people close to narcissists adapt by becoming hyper vigilant to threat or attack. They are always on guard, seeking to anticipate and potentially avoid being in the line of fire. Hypervigilance is emotionally and physiologically debilitating because it drains the body's natural defense system by constantly overloading it. Hypervigilance often leads to Complex Post-Traumatic Stress Disorder (C-PTSD) and illness. Narcissists themselves are hyper vigilant to anything that might trigger their narcissistic injury.

Idealization

Narcissists see the world and others in binary terms – good or bad, black or white. They tend to either idealize or devalue others. Narcissist parents often idealize one golden child and devalue, or scapegoat, others. Their romantic relationships are characterized by a pattern of idealization followed by devaluation and oftentimes discard. When they identify a potential mate, they initially see them as perfect. When the false promise of perfection begins to break down, they cannot see their mate realistically as having a mix of good and flawed qualities. Instead, bitter and punishing disillusionment follows.

Lost Child

This is a child who draws little attention, positive or negative, by staying under the radar and making few demands.

Mascot

This child plays the cute or funny "jester" role, diffusing family tensions without making demands.

Narcissistic Injury

Individuals with Narcissistic Personality Disorder typically suffer an acute and invalidating emotional injury during their early years that interferes with the healthy development of a stable identity and sense of self-esteem. A lack of attunement with caregivers because of loss, rejection, abuse, neglect, or overindulgence (or a messy mix of those things) and a possible genetic predisposition is thought to be at the root of narcissistic injury, leading to foundational feelings of worthlessness. Examples are a child with a mother who dies during his birth and a father who blames him for her death, or a child who is ignored by one parent and habitually praised by the other parent regardless of her efforts or true successes.

Narcissistic Personality Disorder (NPD)

NPD is considered a Cluster B personality disorder defined by the following impairments: overreliance on others for self-definition, overreliance on others for regulation of self-esteem, lack of empathy, exploitative of others, grandiose delusions, exaggerated entitlement, excessive attention seeking, and excessive admiration seeking.

Narcissistic Rage

Narcissistic personalities often react with rage if their narcissist injury is triggered. They take even the smallest slight, which most people would easily brush off, as intense humiliation and/or rejection. When this happens, their fabricated "perfect" self and overblown feelings of entitlement are threatened, setting off a wild rage response. Narcissistic rage is terrifying, sometimes physically violent, and far beyond normal anger. It is emotionally and physically traumatizing for those on the receiving end, particularly children, who naturally blame themselves for adults' reactions.

Narcissistic Supply

People with Narcissistic Personality Disorder depend emotionally on others to sustain their sense of identity and regulate their self-esteem. They get their narcissistic supply either by idealizing and emulating others or by devaluing and asserting their superiority over them. Anyone they can manipulate – a partner, child, friend, or colleague – is a potential source of supply. Without suppliers, narcissists are empty husks. If a source of supply pulls away, they may attempt to hoover them back and/or look for other sources.

Neglect

This is a passive form of abuse in which caregivers ignore the emotional, psychological, and/or physical needs of their dependent(s). It can range from not providing adequate food or shelter to failing to provide affection, supervision, or protection.

No Contact

People who have been abused by a narcissist may choose to cut ties altogether with that person. Typically, people who end up going no contact have had their boundaries violated in traumatic ways that eventually push them to shut down all communication with the narcissist. For adult children of narcissists, going no contact is typically a deeply ambivalent and painful choice that feels like a matter of survival in order to break the cycle of hurt and to attempt to heal. Going no contact, especially from a parent, is difficult to explain to people who don't understand narcissism and its devastating effects, further isolating victims.

NPD

This is the acronym for *Narcissistic Personality Disorder.*

Object Constancy

People with Narcissistic Personality Disorder suffer from a lack of object constancy, or the ability to sustain in real time an awareness of overall positive feelings and past positive experiences with people in their lives when they are disappointed or hurt by them in some way. When triggered, the narcissist's continuity of perception collapses into present-moment reactive emotion. If his child forgets to do a chore, for example, the narcissist father may become enraged and punish him/her, seeing his/her behavior as spiteful or irresponsible even if he/she is usually conscientious.

Parentification

This is a role reversal whereby a parent inappropriately looks to a child, usually the oldest or most capable, to take on parental roles and responsibilities in the family. Narcissists often parentify a child to meet their emotional, physical, and/or sexual needs. Parentification is an extreme violation of children's boundaries, burdening them with adult responsibilities. A parentified child may be expected to play the role of confidante, therapist, or surrogate spouse, as well as perform adult duties, such as caring for younger siblings, cooking, cleaning, managing finances, or earning money for the family.

Projection

Simply put, projection is attributing one's own feelings, actions, or traits onto someone else. Through projection, narcissists blame the victim and deny accountability. If they lie, you are the liar; if they are childish, you are immature; if they insult you, you are critical; if they demand reassurance, you are insecure. Projection is especially traumatic for children, who internalize the belief that they are like their abuser or hurting the person who is actually abusing them. Narcissists also may project their ideal beliefs about themselves onto others, such as their golden child or someone they admire. Narcissists project both consciously and unconsciously.

Scapegoat

This is a child (or children) singled out unfairly for disfavored treatment in the narcissistic family. Scapegoats are typically blamed for family problems, disciplined or punished disproportionately, burdened with excessive chores and responsibilities, and subjected to unmerited negative treatment.

Smear Campaign

Narcissists engage in smear campaigns to discredit others within their family or social sphere. Narcissists may smear another person because that person sees through their mask, they are trying to conceal pre-emptively their own abuse of that person, or they are taking revenge because the person offended or rejected them. Narcissists may conduct a smear campaign for lesser reasons, such as jealousy or resentment. Narcissists can be quite calculating in their process of discrediting and socially isolating their target, using innuendo, gossip, and outright lies to family, friends, neighbors, and community members. Narcissists won't hesitate to smear an ex to their children, a scapegoated child to friends and relatives, or a colleague to other colleagues. The smear campaign usually happens behind the victim's back, often with the assistance of the narcissist's enablers/flying monkeys.

FAQS

1. What's the difference between healthy and extreme narcissism?

Healthy narcissism is all the good points of narcissism, such as a whole bundle of self-confidence and the positive energy to use that to drive you towards success, without any of the negative side effects of it. Someone who has this isn't cut off from the emotional side of life and doesn't put others down to make them feel better. This won't come from anything in childhood, and is actually a desired trait. A bit of self-love can help us all.

Extreme narcissism is the opposite end of the scale. It's narcissism taken as far as it can, to sociopathy and psychopathy. People who suffer from Narcissistic Personality Disorder cannot be helped by someone who isn't medically trained in this area, and it's much better to escape the situation before you get caught up in it yourself.

2. What's an abusive cycle?

An abusive cycle is a continual pattern of negative behavior that doesn't stop no matter what happens. It can be hard to recognize this is what you're in until you take a step back and examine your current situation. It's thought to start with a tension building, then there will be an incident of yelling or maybe violence, then there will be a reconciliation followed by a calm. But the calm never lasts, and the victim is always acutely aware of that.

If this is something you think you might be involved in, then you need to get some emotional support right away. Check out the local abuse resources in your area, because they will be able to point you in the right direction.

3. How can you identify a narcissist?

Working out who is a narcissist early in is a very useful tool because it means you'll be able to identify what's going on before you become consumed by it. Usually, people don't realize what's happening until they are much too embroiled in the situation and cannot extract themselves easily. *Psychology Today* (at www.psychologytoday.com) has presented **five early signs to look out for**:

- Bragging about having a perfect life – no one has that!
- Generosity is a show for others to see, then they are cold at home.
- Imagining rejection and criticism that isn't really happening.
- Experiencing manic emotions, shifting wildly high and low, especially if they don't get what they want.
- Insulting others frequently, especially people they consider beneath themselves.

If all of these sound too familiar, then it might be time to think about what you want your next move to be before you get stuck yourself.

> "Arguing with a NARCISSIST is like getting arrested. Everything you say can and will be used against you."

4. Why was I targeted?

There are many reasons why a narcissist might choose you, but the simplest answer is that you had something that they want. That might be power or beauty, it might be information, or even a vulnerable side that they know they can manipulate. As shown in a previous chapter, you might even have been chosen because you are a challenge, someone who they know they will struggle to manipulate, making it all about the game. It isn't a bad thing that you were targeted, and it doesn't make you weak. More unlucky.

5. What are the signs I need to look out for?

If you believe that you might already be in a relationship with, or are very close to, someone who suffers from narcissism, **you might notice the following things**:

- Wanting to control everything about you; who you see, what you wear, how you act – nothing belongs to you anymore.
- Obsession with how they come across. A constant need to impress everyone else.
- A fragile ego that's easily damaged, often by perceived things rather than something that's actually happened.
- Devaluation of others. The narcissist might quickly become enamored with someone with power, but the slightest provocation can cause them to drop them and despise them.
- No regard for others, especially those seen as below them.
- A history of volatile relationships. If when you first meet them you hear of hundreds of 'crazy exes,' it might be time to worry a little. That isn't good news at all. Don't believe everything you're being told.

STOP!

You cannot effectively communicate with a person that uses emotional reasoning, projection and blame so disengage. When you engage in this level of distress, you will lose control and react emotionally thereby giving the high conflict person the weapon he or she needs to hurt you. By disengaging you will stay in control of your emotions and the high conflict person will lose control.

~Co-parenting With A High Conflict Person~

6. How do I overcome the narcissistic abuse?

You can overcome the abuse you have suffered, but you might not be able to do it alone. The person you really need to work on is yourself. You need to understand the other person, but work on *you* and regain your own strength to help you move past it. A medical professional or therapist will have services to assist you with this. Asking for help is a big, but essential, step to getting control of your own life once more.

7. Where can I get help for a narcissist?

Not every case of narcissism is as clean cut and as easy to walk away from. If the way the other person behaves isn't abuse, then what you might wish to do is help them. *Narcissism Cured* (at https://narcissismcured.com) is an excellent online resource filled with real life stories of people who have suffered from narcissism and recovered. This can help you to see how other people who have been through similar situations have recovered from it. *Medicine Net* (at medicinenet.com/narcissistic_personality_disorder/article.htm) also can help you to find a relevant support group and medical professional in your area.

8. What causes narcissism?

Narcissism is widely thought, by medical professionals who have studied it, to be caused by a difficult childhood. Either neglectful parents or ones who piled on the pressure too much. Something has caused the sufferer to disassociate and deal with their emotions differently. Because of this, there are ways to recover from it, it just takes a lot of willingness and hard work.

Major causes?

- Problems with interpersonal relationships
    - Insensitive – paranoid, psychopathic
    - Demanding – psychopathic, narcissistic
    - Manipulative – Machiavellian
    - Authoritarian – narcissistic, psychopathic, Machiavellian
    - Aloof -- Schizoid
    - Critical – paranoid,
    - Overly cautious – Passive-aggressive, Avoidant
    - Arrogant – Narcissistic!!!
    - Volatile – Histrionic, Borderline
    - Perfectionistic – Obsessive Compulsive
    - Too eager to please – Dependent

CONCLUSION

This book has shown you that narcissism isn't as straightforward as someone being a nasty, selfish person just for the sake of it. Actually, it's often a childhood trauma that's had a negative, lasting impact on the sufferer. Of course, while this doesn't help the victim to recover from the way that they've been treated, it might be a step towards understanding. This understanding can then lead to identifying the behavioral patterns, which, as shown in this book, is the first step to recovering from it, for the perpetrator and the victim.

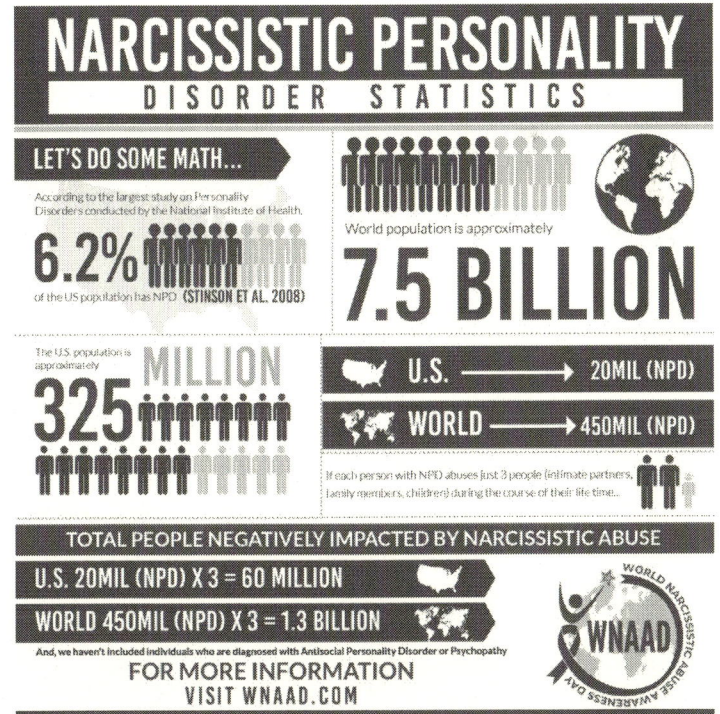

Because narcissism is so common, almost everyone is affected by it in one way or another. Chances are, you *will* encounter someone who suffers from it in your life. These people might be a mild case, in which case you'll hardly notice it, or they might be at the extreme end of the scale, in which case there's a potential for danger, and that's something you need to be very aware of.

A victim of narcissism abuse can use **these steps to begin their road to recovery**:

- Set personal boundaries and stick to them no matter what.
- Rid your life of toxicity. If the perpetrator doesn't want to change, then you need to leave.
- Acknowledge everything that happened and forgive yourself for it. Yes, you knew that you were stuck in an abusive cycle and you should have done something sooner, but you're doing something now!
- Heal yourself. This will take some time, a good look at yourself, and some distance, but it's a very important step if you ever want to fully recover.
- Focus on something else! There's more to life, and now is the time to start looking at it.

The narcissist can also do some work on themselves too, especially if the infliction is only mild. If you fear it might be more towards the extreme side of things, then professional medical assistance is essential. If not, **try these steps**:

- Be aware of the boundaries of others and try to stick to them. This will take some active listening, but can be done. Address people by their names, listen carefully, express interest.
- Always deliver. Don't puff out your chest and promise what you can't do. This will improve your relationships tenfold.
- Think before you act. Take a moment to wonder how your actions might come across to others, then work out if that's a version of yourself that you want to be.
- Get help. This can be support from friends or family, or from someone more professional, but be sure to do it.
- Forgive yourself. Yes, you've made mistakes but you're human. To move forward, you need to forgive what you've done.
- Rebuild your relationships, start engaging in the real world again properly.

There *is* hope. Nothing is a hopeless situation; you just need to work out what is best for yourself. The actionable steps presented in this book should help you to make progress towards getting back to yourself and living a healthy, stress-free life again. Good luck!

ABOUT THE AUTHOR

Lisa Howard is a certified psychotherapist and mental health practitioner who has studied the fields of psychology and sociology. She is considered an expert in the fields of narcissism, gaslighting, trauma treatment, and narcissistic abuse. In this book, she provides a detailed exploration of both her expertise on the subject of narcissism and her personal experiences with narcissistic individuals.

Howard found herself at different points in life closely involved in narcissistic relationships, experiencing firsthand the damage that narcissistic abuse can cause in life and future relationships. Overcoming the trauma caused by these relationships and traveling down the road to recovery herself gave Howard a unique understanding of the difficult path an individual recovering from a narcissistic relationship must follow to recover. The impact of the trauma she experienced influenced the choices she made every day, resulting in a determination to fight and find a powerful way to triumph over her trauma and share her discoveries with others. Howard approaches the subject with empathy and firmness, combining her expertise with her shared experience to create an uncomplicated journey towards recovery.

Made in the USA
Middletown, DE
06 May 2021